Global Perspectives of Employee Assistance Programs

Global Perspectives of Employee Assistance Programs is the first book of its kind to empirically address the Employee Assistance Program (EAP) concept and model in a diverse, global context. This book features a variety of studies which deal with the design, delivery, cultural adaptability, evaluation, and measurement of international employee assistance programs in a truly global variety of settings. Contributors also evaluate the impact of EAP on expatriates, the potential for an international well-being assessment tool, and the training of international EAP professionals.

This book was originally published as a special issue of the *Journal of Workplace Behavioral Health*.

R. Paul Maiden is Executive Vice Dean and Professor in the School of Social Work, at the University of Southern California, Los Angeles, USA. The USC School of Social Work is a top-ranked program and the largest graduate school of social work in the United States. He brings 30 years of expertise to the field of workplace human services. He is the past Editor-in-Chief (2000–2015) of the *Journal of Workplace Behavioral Health*, the only peer-reviewed journal in employee assistance research and practice. He is the recipient of two Senior Fulbright Scholar awards to Russia and South Africa that focused on development of workplace programs.

David A. Sharar is Managing Director of Chestnut Global Partners (CGP), Bloomington, Illinois, USA, a provider of domestic and international employee assistance, expatriate support, and crisis intervention. His passion is to help CGP's international provider partners adapt the 'western' behavioral health and EAP concepts to fit local cultural contexts, as well as building the organizational capability to innovate, execute, and measure results.

Global Perspectives of Employee Assistance Programs

Edited by
R. Paul Maiden and David A. Sharar

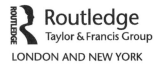

Routledge
Taylor & Francis Group

LONDON AND NEW YORK

First published 2016 by Routledge

2 Park Square, Milton Park, Abingdon, Oxfordshire OX14 4RN
711 Third Avenue, New York, NY 10017

Routledge is an imprint of the Taylor & Francis Group, an informa business

First issued in paperback 2017

British Library Cataloguing in Publication Data
A catalogue record for this book is available from the British Library

ISBN 13: 978-1-138-96265-1 (hbk)
ISBN 13: 978-1-138-30242-6 (pbk)

Typeset in Garamond
by RefineCatch Limited, Bungay, Suffolk

Publisher's Note
The publisher accepts responsibility for any inconsistencies that may have arisen during the conversion of this book from journal articles to book chapters, namely the possible inclusion of journal terminology.

Disclaimer
Every effort has been made to contact copyright holders for their permission to reprint material in this book. The publishers would be grateful to hear from any copyright holder who is not here acknowledged and will undertake to rectify any errors or omissions in future editions of this book.

Contents

CONTENTS

Citation Information

The chapters in this book were originally published in the *Journal of Workplace Behavioral Health*, volume 30, issues 1–2 (Jan–June 2015). When citing this material, please use the original page numbering for each article, as follows:

Chapter 1
First Nations, Maori, American Indians, and Native Hawaiians as Sovereigns: EAP with Indigenous Nations Within Nations
Rodney C. Haring, Māui Hudson, Louisa Erickson, Maile Taualii, and Bonnie Freeman
Journal of Workplace Behavioral Health, volume 30, issues 1–2 (Jan–June 2015) pp. 14–31

Chapter 2
Employee Assistance Programs in Australia: Evaluating Success
Robert-Leigh Compton and John G. McManus
Journal of Workplace Behavioral Health, volume 30, issues 1–2 (Jan–June 2015) pp. 32–45

Chapter 3
Using an Interactive Self-Assessment Tool to Strengthen Your Employee Assistance Service
Liliana Dias, Audrey Eertmans, Inge Van den Brande, Yasmin Handaja, Sofie Taeymans, and Debora Vansteenwegen
Journal of Workplace Behavioral Health, volume 30, issues 1–2 (Jan–June 2015) pp. 46–65

Chapter 4
Evaluating EAP Counseling in the Chinese Workplace: A Study with a Brief Instrument
Peizhong Li, David A. Sharar, Richard Lennox, and Wei Zhuang
Journal of Workplace Behavioral Health, volume 30, issues 1–2 (Jan–June 2015) pp. 66–78

Chapter 5
Eureka: An Employee Services Perception Study in Continental Europe
Debora Vansteenwegen, Manuel Sommer, Dirk Antonissen, Tito Laneiro, and Odete Nunes
Journal of Workplace Behavioral Health, volume 30, issues 1–2 (Jan–June 2015) pp. 79–111

Chapter 6

Innovative Career Support Services for Professional Women in India: Pathways to Success
Beverly Younger, Kalpana Tatavarti, Neeti Poorswani, Denica Gordon-Mandel,
Caitlin Hannon, Ikiah K. McGowan, and Gokul Mandayam
Journal of Workplace Behavioral Health, volume 30, issues 1–2 (Jan–June 2015) pp. 112–137

Chapter 7

A Substance Abuse Intervention Program at a Large Russian Manufacturing Worksite
Kenneth Burgess, Richard Lennox, David A. Sharar, and Alexander Shtoulman
Journal of Workplace Behavioral Health, volume 30, issues 1–2 (Jan–June 2015)
pp. 138–153

Chapter 8

*Pricing Models of Employee Assistance Programs: Experiences of Corporate Clients Serviced by
a Leading Employee Assistance Program Service Provider in South Africa*
Neliswa A. Cekiso and Lourens S. Terblanche
Journal of Workplace Behavioral Health, volume 30, issues 1–2 (Jan–June 2015)
pp. 154–178

Chapter 9

*The Effects of Psychosocial Problems on Employees' Stress, Self-Esteem, and Organizational
Commitment: The Case of South Korean Workplaces*
Soochan Choi, Jeongeun Lee, and Haewoong Park
Journal of Workplace Behavioral Health, volume 30, issues 1–2 (Jan–June 2015)
pp. 179–190

Chapter 10

*Response to the Challenge of Training International EAP Professionals: An Online Certificate
Program*
Dale A. Masi and Kent Carlson
Journal of Workplace Behavioral Health, volume 30, issues 1–2 (Jan–June 2015)
pp. 191–208

Chapter 11

*Group Characteristics and Mental Health of Chinese Expatriates in Africa and Central Asia:
A Multisite, Multiyear Study*
Peizhong Li, David A. Sharar, and Jie Zhang
Journal of Workplace Behavioral Health, volume 30, issues 1–2 (Jan–June 2015)
pp. 209–227

For any permission-related enquiries please visit:
http://www.tandfonline.com/page/help/permissions

Notes on Contributors

Dirk Antonissen has an academic background in Psychology and Finance, and since 2000 he has been the CEO of ISW Limits, a spin-off company of Leuven University, Belgium. ISW Limits is active in the field of EAP and introduces innovative approaches and tools in this field. Since 2007, he has also been a board member of the Employee Assistance European Forum, and a (keynote) speaker at many international conferences. Before 2000, he worked as a team leader, a chief technical advisor, and a management consultant for international projects.

Kenneth Burgess is a rehabilitation counsellor with more than 30 years of international experience. A graduate of the University of Pittsburgh, PA, USA, he began his career as an occupational alcoholism professional for US Steel in Pennsylvania, then served as the EAP manager for two Fortune 500 organizations: Gulf Oil and Alcoa. He began his own company in 1998, Solutions, Latin America, an EAP based in Sao Paulo, Brazil. He has also lived and worked as an expatriate in Australia and Russia.

Kent Carlson is a Technology Associate for Masi Research Consultants, Inc., and Program Coordinator for the Massachusetts Department of Conservation and Recreation. He is a technology business analyst and consultant implementing effective solutions for people, systems, and processes.

Neliswa A. Cekiso currently holds the position of Deputy Director in the National Department of Social Development (South Africa) as Manager of Social Work Policy. Her Master's research topic 'Pricing Models of Employee Assistance Programs: Experiences of Corporate Clients Serviced by a Leading Employee Assistance Program Service Provider in South Africa' culminated in the development of a guideline that could be applied to inform practice in pricing models. Her areas of work include provision of support to provincial departments of social development, civil society, and other national departments to enhance work productivity in the field of child protection.

Soochan Choi is a Professor in the Department of Social Welfare, and Associate Dean of the College of Social Science, at Yonsei University, Seoul, South Korea, where he specializes in occupational social work. He is also a member of the Board of Directors of the Korea Employee Assistance Professionals Association (KEAPA).

Robert-Leigh Compton is Conjoint Associate Professor in the Newcastle Business School within the University of Newcastle, Australia. He has previously worked as National Head of the Business School at ACU National, as Foundation Director of Academic Programs at the

Sydney Graduate School of Management, and MBA Director at the University of Western Sydney. He has co-authored five editions of *Effective Recruitment and Selection Practices*, and seven editions (with Dr. Alan Nankervis) of *Strategic Human Resource Management*.

Liliana Dias is currently pursuing a PhD in Psychology at the University of Leuven, Belgium. She holds a Masters in Psychology from the University of Lisbon, Portugal. Professionally, she works as a business unit manager at a local EAP provider company based in Lisbon, Portugal (outCOme – Clínica Organizacional, Lda.). She has been working in the field of EAP since 2006.

Audrey Eertmans is Senior Project and Account Manager at ISW Limits and European Branch Office Manager of Chestnut Global Partners. At ISW Limits, she has been responsible for the project 'Stress at Work' (2000–2007), ordered and funded by the European Social Fund (ESF). Today, she manages accounts in various economic sectors, supporting and guiding companies in the development and implementation of integrated programs related to well-being at work, including surveys, ISAT, training, and EAP. At CGP, she manages accounts in Western Europe and collaborates with the Division of Commercial Science.

Louisa Erickson is a member of the Whakatōhea tribe on the Eastern Coast of the North Island in New Zealand. She has been the Iwi Social Services Manager for the Whakatōhea Māori Trust Board since 2009 and has management experience in both the health and education sectors. She loves living at home, and her wish is that her children will one day return to Opotiki with all of her grandchildren. She believes this is their homeland and wants them to work and contribute to the exciting future that exists for Whakatōhea.

Bonnie Freeman is an Algonquin/Mohawk from the Six Nations of the Grand River Territory in Ontario, Canada. Her doctoral degree is in Social Work from Wilfrid Laurier University, Waterloo, Canada. She is currently a Lecturer at McMaster University, Hamilton, Canada, which will soon transition to a tenure-track assistant professorship in the School of Social Work. She brings many years of practice experience, as well as experience as a course instructor for several post-secondary institutions.

Denica Gordon-Mandel is a registered psychological assistant for the Beverly Hills, California health group Cognitive Behavior Associates, under the supervision of Dr. Joel L. Becker. She has more than 15 years of work experience in marketing communications within both the public and private sectors, specializing in organization positioning, issues management, internal and external communications, as well as crisis communications. She utilizes her professional and clinical skills to provide individuals and organizations interventions that increase behavioural health and effectiveness. She specializes in women's wellness, stress management, diversity issues, and leadership development.

Yasmin Handaja holds a master's degree in Work and Occupational Psychology from the University of Leuven, Belgium. After obtaining her master's degree, she continued working at the university, conducting scientific research in the domain of quantitative and qualitative job insecurity within the context of restructuring, and its influence on psychosocial well-being of employees. Since 2007, she has been the Head of Surveys & Assessments at ISW Limits. In this capacity, she offers consultancy and guidance to companies within various economic sectors in the development of an integrated policy on motivation, engagement, and well-being at work.

Caitlin Hannon is a recent graduate from the School of Social Work at the University of Southern California, Los Angeles, CA, USA, where she specialized in Social Work and Business in a Global Society. She is currently working as a human resources professional in the entertainment industry where she pursues her interests which include innovative approaches to employee engagement and work life management.

Rodney C. Haring is the Founder of One Feather Consulting, a joint venture company with Chestnut Global Partners. As a majority Native American-owned entity, the firm offers culturally-attuned comprehensive EAP, work/life, and disease management services worldwide specifically designed for Indigenous workforces, communities, and landscapes. He is a Nation Congress of American Indians scholar, past Fellow of the Spirit of EAGLES Program at the Mayo Clinic, and a former Robert Wood Johnson Foundation New Connections Grantee. Dr. Haring (Beaver Clan) is an enrolled member of the Seneca Nation of Indians and resides on the Cattaraugus Indian Reservation with his family. In 2010, he was an expert panel member to the United States Department of Education, the White House Office of National Drug Control Policy, Executive Office to the President. His research interests include various health disparities that are prevalent within Native American societies with a special interest in cancer and obesity.

Māui Hudson is from Whakatōhea, Ngā Ruahine and Te Mahurehure. He is a Research Developer and Interdisciplinary Researcher based at the University of Waikato, New Zealand. He holds Senior Research Fellow positions within the Māori and Indigenous Governance Centre in the Faculty of Law and the Environmental Research Institute in the Faculty of Science and Engineering. He has worked in the research sector for over 10 years in both CRI and university settings, is a member of the Whakatōhea Māori Trust Board, and a director on a tribal health and social service company. He has a diverse range of research interests in the area of the interface between mātauranga Māori and science, ethics and new technologies, traditional medicine, and Māori economic development.

Tito Laneiro is a Psychologist and Professor at Lisbon Autonomous University, Portugal, where he is the scientific coordinator of the bachelor's degree in Psychology, member of the Pedagogic Council of the University, and a member of the Psychology Research Centre CIP-UAL. He coordinates the New Work Research Group (NWRG). Besides being the author of several scientific articles, he is a specialist in Organizational Psychology. He has also been an organizational consultant for many years.

Jeongeun Lee obtained her master's and doctoral degrees in Social Work from Yonsei University, Seoul, South Korea. She currently works as a Senior Researcher at Seoul National University Hospital, where she has conducted a series of research projects on rehabilitation services and healthcare access for people with disabilities. Her research interests are in the areas of work-family balance and EAP effectiveness, as well as disability and health inequality.

Richard Lennox holds a doctoral degree from Texas Tech University, Lubbock, TX, USA, in Experimental Social Psychology. He began his working career at the Institute for Research in Social Science at the University of North Carolina, Chapel Hill, NC, USA. Since then, he has been largely employed as a statistician and methodologist at contract research organizations. He is currently the Chief Scientist and Vice President of Commercial Science at Chestnut Global Partners, in Chestnut Health Systems. It was at Chestnut that he developed the Workplace Outcomes Suite (WOS) as a scientifically validated measure of EAP effectiveness that is widely used throughout the industry.

Peizhong Li has served as a Senior Researcher at Chestnut Global Partners, China, since 2012. His expertise in Employee Assistance Programs includes mental health assessment, program evaluation, and training. After receiving his doctoral degree in Psychology in the United States, he held teaching and research positions at the University of Wisconsin-Stout, USA, and Hohai University, Nanjing, China, for seven years. He has published research papers in social psychology in international peer-reviewed journals.

R. Paul Maiden is Executive Vice Dean and Professor in the School of Social Work, at the University of Southern California, Los Angeles, USA. The USC School of Social Work is a top-ranked program and the largest graduate school of social work in the United States. He brings 30 years of expertise to the field of workplace human services. He is the past Editor-in-Chief (2000–2015) of the *Journal of Workplace Behavioral Health*, the only peer-reviewed journal in employee assistance research and practice. He is the recipient of two Senior Fulbright Scholar awards to Russia and South Africa that focused on development of workplace programs.

Gokul Mandayam is a Clinical Associate Professor and a member of the community organization, planning and administration (COPA) concentration in the School of Social Work at the University of Southern California, Los Angeles, CA, USA. He has worked as an evaluation consultant for both public and non-profit sectors, as well as a qualitative market researcher for the corporate sector. His interdisciplinary research interests include applications of geographic information systems technology for human services, international social development, program evaluation, and public and non-profit management. His teaching focuses on the provision of research-based and technological solutions to address the problems of society, organizations, and individuals, and enhancement of knowledge on the public policy process to assist social workers in their macro practice endeavours.

Dale A. Masi is Professor Emeritus at the University of Maryland, College Park, MD, USA. She is President and CEO of Masi Research Consultants, Inc., a Boston, USA, company specializing in EAP evaluation. She is the author of 15 books and more than 70 articles dealing with EAPs. She is a Fulbright Scholar and has consulted in 45 countries for the US State Department and other international organizations. She is a NASW Social Work Pioneer in Employee Assistance.

Ikiah K. McGowan is a recent graduate of the Masters of Social Work program at the University of Southern California, Los Angeles, CA, USA, where she concentrated on Social Work and Business in a Global Society. She has professional experience in multiple industries, such as advertising, finance, politics, and entertainment. Her interests lie in the collaboration between businesses, non-profit organizations, and passionate individuals to facilitate social impact in the form of conscious capitalism, corporate social responsibility, and cause marketing. She is applying her expertise as a philanthropy consultant for Fortune 500 companies and start up organizations.

John G. McManus is the current President of EAPAA, which is the peak body for EAP professionals in Australia and New Zealand. He is the Chair of the Ethics committee and regularly consults on what constitutes good and ethical practice. He is a partner and senior psychologist in Mind & Matter Consulting, which is a consulting firm involved in the provision of EAPs to numerous corporations and not-for-profit entities as well as a range of other psychological services. His PhD thesis focused on the psychoanalytic study of organizations and established that EAPs do provide significant health benefits to employees and their families. He has worked in the field of EAPs for over 25 years and is highly committed to the promotion of health and well-being.

Odete Nunes is a PCE accredited psychotherapist and trainer in Leader Effectiveness Training, Teacher Effectiveness Training, and Parents Effectiveness Training with Gordon Training International; Director of the Psychology and Sociology Department of Universidade Autónoma de Lisboa, Portugal; and scientific coordinator of the Psychology Research Centre CIP-UAL.

Haewoong Park is Chief Manager of the toll business policy team at the Korea Expressway Corporation. As HR Manager in his prior position, he has promoted various corporate welfare programs, such as employee assistance programs, work/life solutions, and wellness programs. From labour's perspectives, he has also conducted valuable studies on corporate welfare in order to improve the quality of working life in South Korea.

Neeti Poorswani is a Principal Consultant at Interweave Consulting. She brings diverse experiences and skills from across a variety of sectors. Through her work in the non-profit and development sector, she has developed holistic expertise across issues of gender, child rights, formal and non-formal education, and social constructs. Over the past five years, she has worked in a variety of roles at Interweave, from content development, delivery, and training, to managing various diversity events and conferences.

David A. Sharar is Managing Director of Chestnut Global Partners (CGP), Bloomington, Illinois, USA, a provider of domestic and international employee assistance, expatriate support, and crisis intervention. His passion is to help CGP's international provider partners adapt the 'western' behavioral health and EAP concepts to fit local cultural contexts, as well as building the organizational capability to innovate, execute, and measure results.

Alexander Shtoulman graduated from First Moscow Medical University, Russia, as a General Physician in 1972. Since then, his professional experience moved him to the field of cardiology, resuscitation, and emergency medicine. Since 1990, his education and practice has been in the field of addiction counselling, one of the first in Russia. With growing expertise in the addictions field, he worked on the design of an educational program for addiction specialists in Moscow Municipal University of Psychology and Pedagogue, Russia. Acknowledging the need for new, effective approaches to managing different kinds of destructive human behavior, he works to introduce Employee Assistance Services to Russian employers and employees.

Manuel Sommer is the founder and Director of Clinica CAPA in Lisbon, Portugal. Coming originally from the addiction treatment field, where he has worked in Portugal, Switzerland, the UK, and Brazil, he has become more and more involved in Employee Assistance work and EAPs, having pioneered this field in Portugal. With over 20 years of experience working with clients and organizations in several clinical and organizational issues and settings, he currently works as a consultant and trainer and is an Associate Professor of Psychology at the Autonomous University in Lisbon, Portugal, where he is also a Senior Researcher in the Psychology Research Centre.

Sofie Taeymans has over 10 years of experience in conducting applied research at ISW Limits NV, a spin-off company of the University of Leuven, Belgium. In her current position as Senior Product Development Manager, she focuses on developing and validating instruments and applying them in innovative online (self-)assessment environments. She is co-author of several publications on the validation of questionnaires in the field of well-being at work, such as stress and motivation, work-related worrying and safety.

Kalpana Tatavarti is a partner at Interweave Consulting Pvt Ltd, providing training, facilitating, and executive coaching. As a founder at Maarpidi, a learning and development firm, she partnered with several organizations to grow their leadership pipelines. A passionate crusader of inclusive workplaces, she heads the Women's Leadership Development vertical and has worked closely with many organizations to grow their female leaders. She credits her deep understanding of gender in the Indian workplace to the 1500 women managers she has trained and coached across the country. She shares this understanding with leaders and managers in her Gender Sensitization & Prevention of Sexual Harassment interventions.

Maile Taualii is an Assistant Professor and Chair of Native Hawaiian and Indigenous Health at the University of Hawai'i, USA, where she brings cultural, ethical, and community-oriented perspectives to the instruction of public health. Her primary research focus is the utility and validity of health information for racial minorities, and her current research is related to perceptions of bio-banking for research among Native Hawaiians. Her federal commitments include serving as a member of the National Advisory Committee on Racial, Ethnic, and Other Populations, US Census Bureau, and co-Chairing the Regional Health Equity Council, Department of Health and Human Service, Office of Minority Health.

Lourens S. Terblanche holds a doctorate in Social Work and is an Associate Professor at the University of Pretoria, South Africa. He has published in a number of journals and presented papers at a number of national and international conferences. He specializes in social work supervision and management as well as Employee Assistance Programs, and is the program manager for the master's program in EAPs, actively involved in continuing education, research, national and international structures in the EAP field. He was the President of the Employee Assistance Professionals Association of South Africa from 2009 to 2011. He was awarded 'Exceptional EAP Professional' in September 2011 by the Employee Assistance Professionals Association of South Africa. In 2002, he received the 'Special Recognition Award' from EAPA, and in October 2012 he was awarded 'EAPA Member of the Year' by the Employee Assistance Professionals Association for his contribution to the enhancement of Employee Assistance Programs both nationally and internationally.

Inge Van den Brande holds a PhD in Human Resource Management from Leuven University, Belgium. After obtaining her PhD, she continued working at the University as a Scientific Researcher in the domain of HR and Organizational Behavior (psychological contract, job and organizational commitment, employee motivation, competence management). She has also been Professor in Human Resource Management at Leuven University. Since 2007, she has worked as a Senior Project and Account Manager at ISW Limits. Her main responsibility is assisting companies in the set-up of a policy on well-being and engagement, with the help of different tools and methodologies developed by ISW Limits.

Debora Vansteenwegen was Research Director of ISW Limits, a spinoff company of Leuven University, Belgium, and Senior Postdoctoral Researcher in the Department of Psychology of the University of Leuven. She has published widely on the topics of fear and anxiety disorders, their etiology, and treatment. Her current activities focus on e-mental health, positive psychology, well-being at work, employee assistance, and stress management programs. She has more than 10 years of experience in coordinating research projects, advising, and stimulating innovative research and the development of instruments and tools for applications in HRM and well-being policy at work.

Beverly Younger is a Clinical Associate Professor and the Chair of the Social Work and Business in a Global Society concentration in the School of Social Work at the University of Southern California, Los Angeles, CA, USA. She worked extensively in the role of Employee Assistance manager and consultant with both manufacturing and services businesses. Her work later transitioned into organizational development, program design and evaluation, and facilitation and training for public, private, and governmental organizations, with an emphasis on organizational and personal empowerment. Her research interests and publications have focused on corporate responses to the personal needs of workers and to federal legislation regulating employer personnel practices. Her current research projects examine global perspectives on corporate social responsibility and career support services for women.

Jie Zhang has served as the General Manager of Chestnut Global Partners, China, since its establishment in 2005. Over the last decade she has overseen the creation and development of Chestnut Global Partners' employee assistance programs in China, building comprehensive operations serving more than 250,000 employees at local and multinational companies today.

Wei Zhuang is currently employed by PscyCN-Chestnut Global Partners in Beijing, China, where she is a research specialist. During employment at PCGP, she has been involved in a series of research projects on employees' well-being. She is pursuing a PhD in Industrial and Organizational Psychology at the University at Albany, NY, USA.

First Nations, Maori, American Indians, and Native Hawaiians as Sovereigns: EAP with Indigenous Nations Within Nations

RODNEY C. HARING, PhD, MSW

One Feather Consulting, Cattaraugus Territory of the Seneca Nation; Office of Health Disparities, Cancer Prevention, and Population Sciences, Roswell Park Cancer Institute, Buffalo, New York, USA

MĀUI HUDSON, BHSc AIT, MHSc AUT

Te Piringa Faculty of Law, University of Waikato, Hamilton, New Zealand

LOUISA ERICKSON

Whakatōhea Māori Trust Board, Ōpōtiki, New Zealand

MAILE TAUALII, PhD, MPH

Native Hawaiian and Indigenous Health at the University of Hawai'i, Honolulu, Hawai'i, USA

BONNIE FREEMAN, PhD(c), MSW

School of Social Work, McMaster University, Hamilton, Ontario, Canada

Indigenous workforces have existed across the world since the creation of Earth. What has changed is the evolution of multicultural societies, governments, and landscapes that have become part of, or sit parallel to, sovereign Indigenous nations and their workforces. An international response to Employee Assistance Programming (EAP) and workplace health will be shared from various Indigenous groups across the globe. These societies include the Maori of New Zealand, First Nations of Canada, American Indian groups from the U.S. mainland, and Native Hawaiians. Guidelines for EAP practice include the discussion of historical trauma, communication skills, confidentiality, and environmental issues. Theoretical underpinnings for health sovereignty are shared through ancient teachings of Indigenous philosophies and their relationships to contemporary EAP development and utilization.

INTRODUCTION

Long before the Europeans arrived in North America thousands of distinct Indigenous groups inhabited much of North America. The same is true about New Zealand and in the remote Islands of the Pacific where Polynesians settled the main island groups hundreds of years before the arrival of European sailors. Today these societies are known in many different ways: *Native Americans, American Indians, Native Hawaiians, First Nations, tribes,* or *bands.* Due to a variety of historical occurrences roughly 1,000 distinct federally recognized Indigenous Nations exist today in North America, more than 100 distinct *iwi* (tribal entities) in New Zealand. There are also continued negotiations among Indigenous Peoples, such as the Native Hawaiians, whose land is illegally occupied, creating a unique relationship between the Indigenous Peoples of Hawaiʻi and the United States (Public Law 103–150). These Indigenous Nations are sovereign entities within their respective landscape and have long-standing government-to-government relationships as such.

HISTORICAL INDIGENOUS VALUES AND PURPOSE

One distinction related to a value system is the interdependence between individuals and society (Brieland, 1977). A narrative account representing this property stated, "the chiefs are generally the poorest among them, for instead of their receiving from the common peoples as among the Christians, they are obliged to give to the mob" (Megapolensis, as cited in Jamerson, 1909, p. 46). In this passage, the value of sharing is exhibited when individuals in Haudenosaunee society with great power, such as chiefs, relinquish personal items for the betterment of people and society. Barbara General (personal communication, March 1, 2004), RSW (Beaver Clan) of the Six Nations Reserve in Ontario, Canada, indicated that this notion of giving is represented by the Haudensoaunee term *O gwa deni:deo* that translated forms the meaning of "taking care of your own."

A second property of Indigenous value incorporated into Employee Assistance Programming (EAP) practice revolves around the concept of having social responsibility for one another and the responsibility of providing ways to overcome obstacles that cause disequilibrium between individual and environment (Brieland, 1977). An anonymous Dutch writer cited in Van Meteren (1535–1612) wrote the following account:

> We went another league and a half and came to a hunter's cabin, which we entered to eat some venison . . . a chief invited us into his castle. There was a big fire lighted, and a fat haunch of venison cooked, of which we ate. He gave us two bearskins to sleep upon, and presented me with three beaver skins . . . . We slept in this house, ate heartily of pumpkins, beans and venison, so that we were not hungry, but were treated as well as possible in their land. (Jamerson, 1909, p. 141)

In this passage, an Indigenous confederacy of tribes (Haudenosaunee/ Iroquois) presented a historical foundation of social responsibility in the form of food sharing, in this case, across racial boundaries. Another narrative by a Scottish physician, Cadwallader Colden (as cited in McIntosh, 1844), replicated these findings by stating:

> The hospitality of these Indians is no less remarkable than their other virtues. As soon as any stranger comes among them, they are sure to offer him victuals; if a number arrive, one of their best houses is cleaned for their accommodation. (p. 269)

Not only food sharing, but also the sharing of home, residence, and hospitality were features of Haudenosaunee social responsibility as it relates to values. As shared by Merle Watt, Jr. (personal communication, March 1, 2004), a Seneca (Bear Clan) from the Allegany Indian Reservation (USA), "It is the value of sharing and social responsibility that made the Haudenosaunee quite possibly the first North American people without a homeless population."

Foundational EAP practice in the area of purpose focuses on identifying potential areas of disequilibrium between individuals or groups and the environment to prevent the occurrence of disequilibrium (Brieland, 1977). An example of this historical Indigenous property of EAP practice was brought forth by Parker (1913) when he related:

> the Creator states it is a great wrong to be unkind to our grandmothers. He designed that an old woman should be as a child again and when she becomes so the Creator wishes the grandchildren to help her, for only because she is, they are. (p. 13)

This passage conveys that people must realize that keeping a positive process of respect between young and old is of great importance. By highlighting the purpose of care and help for the elderly by her next generation of kin, a cyclical process of positive equilibrium and family cohesion is accomplished. This equilibrium is accomplished in part by the purpose of family responsibility. *Family responsibility* is defined as a circle of family care. Although elders care for children as the children mature to keep equilibrium in the family structure, children must care for elders when their health wanes. If compared to modern day EAP practice, by not identifying and acting upon this circle of family care—workplace, social and community equilibrium is at risk.

Social work methods, often used in EAP practice, are described as the responsible, conscious, disciplined use of self in a relationship with an individual or group (Brieland, 1977). One method based in Indigenous philosophy is found in Caldwallader Colden's following narrative account: "they (Haudenosaunee) never execute their resolutions by force upon any of their people. Honour and esteem are their principal rewards; as shame and being despised their punishments" (as cited in McIntosh, 1844, p. 266). This process of disciplinary methodology indicates a nonviolent approach to societal peace. Through the use of psychological punishment in the form of shame and psychological praise in the form of honor and esteem, non-violent methods of group and society balance were promoted.

HEALTH SOVEREIGNTY THROUGH EAP

Sovereignty is described as the right to govern your own direction, a separate entity with self-determined laws, codes, policies, structures, and licensing. Sovereignty has been exercised in many forms in contemporary history. Examples include the use of sovereign status for the development of gaming enterprises. Dr. Donald Warne (Lakota) (personal communication, October 22, 2013), the first Native American candidate for the U.S. Surgeon General, indicated that "sovereignty has been put forward in such initiatives in health care such as the utilization of Indian Health Service health care in the US though the '638 programs' in which tribes have the sovereign ability to structure health care services within their own communities as well as new provisions and set asides in the Affordable Health Care Act where money is specifically designated for federally recognized tribal governments. Hence, Indigenous groups as sovereign entities of their respective landscape have the means to guide their own process of living, well-being, and behavioral health."

In relation to EAP practice, sovereign Indigenous groups have the unique ability to build EAP programs through in-house mechanisms, contract for service, or develop a hybrid model of care. EAPs are designed to provide employees and the employee's family a professional and confidential resource that can be used to address various social, mental, emotional, and health care concerns. These include coworker conflict, stress, substance misuse, marital distress, trauma, and other issues that may affect the individual, family, or community (Haring, 2011).

Although many Indigenous communities offer prevention programs that educate Indigenous peoples on issues of diabetes, obesity, depression, heart disease, and stroke, the resources and support to sustain a healthier lifestyles related to work/life balances are lacking. As a result, rates of chronic disease among Indigenous people continue to rise (Health Canada, 2003; MacMillan, MacMillan, Offord, & Dingle, 1996; Shewell, 2004) leading to increased health disparities among Indigenous employees and the communities they reside in. According to the Statistical Profile on the Health of First Nations in Canada report (Health Canada, 2003), Indigenous people younger than age 30 years make up more than one half of the total Indigenous population. As the population of Indigenous people continues to increase, so do many of the issues, which eventually transcend into the work environment. The report by the Royal Commission on Aboriginal People (Government of Canada, 1996) describes how Indigenous people are going through a loss of cultural identity, high rates of poverty, limited employment opportunities, inadequate living conditions, weakened social structures, and ongoing racism. For many Indigenous employees, these demoralizing conditions have contributed to increased substance abuse, suicide, violence, and mortality (Chandler & Lalonde, 1998; Freeman, 2004; Olson & Wahab, 2006; Strickland, Walsh, & Cooper, 2006; White Bear, 2003;).

Another growing concern within Indigenous communities is the usage of methamphetamines. Studies show rates of methamphetamines use of 1.7% for U.S. Indigenous populations and 2.2% for Native Hawaiians compared to rates in Whites (0.7%), Hispanics (0.5%), Asians (0.2%), and African-Americans (0.1%) (Office of Applied Studies, 2005). In fact, the National Indian Child Welfare Association estimated that 80% to 85% of the Indigenous families in child welfare systems have drug or alcohol abuse issues (The National Congress of American Indians, 2006).

Evolving and comprehensive approaches in EAP are starting to diversify their offerings to include health coaching, disease management, legal guidance, and financial consultations among other core features. Offerings often include detailed quarterly reports; outcomes-based evaluations of program functioning, encouragement of face-to-face sessions, and on-site crisis management. EAP services are often based on an assessment, short-term counseling, and referral type model which focus on workforce performance and improvement.

INDIGENOUS THEORY: HAUDENOSAUNEE UNDERPINNING SETTING THE STAGE FOR EAP PRACTICE

Since the beginning of time, Indigenous groups have been instructed to strive for peace as individuals, communities, and Nations and to constantly strive to speak, work, live, and to carry on in a peaceful way or mind-set. To the

Haudenosaunee, peace is more than just the absence of conflict but is founded on spiritual and social foundations of wellness. *Peace* has been defined as the active work toward establishing universal justice. True peace is the product of a unified society on the path of good will and good thought through the process of reasoning.

This process of Indigenous theory has a definitive place in the EAP practice and workplace health. When EAP practice works for peace, practitioners have the ability to develop a "good mind" or a "good way of thinking." This "good mind" occurs when an organization(s) and EAP professional incorporate or blend their minds and emotions in harmony with the flow of the intent of wellness in the workplace and the realization of Indigenous space where the intervention occurs. Further, principles related to the "good mind" also encourage that thoughts of prejudice, privilege, or superiority be put to aside and that recognition be given to the reality that the EAP in its capacity of wellness and good intention is designed for the benefit of all equally.

Lastly, the underpinnings of workplace health through the Haudenosaunee lens shapes a workplace with the help of the EAP to work for peace and a good mind and by doing so the EAP within the Indigenous community will develop strength. This strength is then encouraged by strength-based and resiliency focused EAP programming that uses a good mind to incorporate rational thinking and persuasion to channel the inherent good will of the EAP professional to work toward peace, justice and unity to prevent, encourage, promote empowerment, and find resiliency in workplace and community. These concepts of peace, strength and the "good mind" are cited from the protocol for the review of scientific research proposals on territories of the Seneca Nation of Indians (2011) that cited with permission from the Akwesasne Task Force on the Environment Research Advisory Committee (1996).

EAP: MODERN-DAY INDIGENOUS LANDSCAPES

Cultural appropriateness is an ethical factor that underlies EAP practice with any group. However, Indigenous peoples have structures of belief, customs, and historical experiences vastly different from that of EAP professionals trained in mainstream universities. Special care needs to be taken when these same EAP providers or affiliates attempt to apply techniques to Indigenous peoples and within sovereign Indigenous communities.

It is sometimes the case that outside EAP professionals may be viewed negatively in the Indigenous landscape. Indigenous groups have often been exploited, not just by governments and corporations, but also by "Western" researchers who have come in from the outside to study Indigenous people. Often, these sovereign nation communities have not been informed of the study findings nor experienced any benefits of the research. Other instances include information being lost or used in an unethical manner. That being said, EAP professionals work in diverse settings and are exposed to employees, families, and communities in a wealth of circumstances, from children of employees to spouses and elder care givers.

EAP professionals take pride in being able to maneuver assessment, short-term problem solving, and referral skills toward EAP practice understanding as it relates to varying cultures. Sections of this article have been adapted from a previous publication developed for the National Association of Social Work (Haring, 2009) and focuses on background information, environmental contexts, communication skills, and a historical overview for EAP professionals to consider when working with Indigenous employees, families, and societies. Part of EAP practice is comprehending that EAP professionals can never be entirely knowledgeable in any given area, topic, or population. The employee in essence is the true expert on her or his life and its relationship to the workplace. Becoming knowledgeable about cultures and peoples is an ongoing process of keeping an open mind and being receptive to learning, applying, educating in a creative fashion.

EAP Practice Guidelines for Working with Indigenous Employees and Families

This account has been adapted to fit a Haudenosaunee framework from other stories shared by Indigenous groups around the globe. As the story goes, a beaver was interested in crossing the creek to find a new area of twigs, saplings, trees, and other shrubs to eat and to use to build her dam. However, she noticed the creek was very fast. The current was very strong, and beaver had a difficult and challenging time reaching the other side. While making her way across, beaver went under the water several times and nearly ran out of air. When she finally reached the bank, she fainted from exhaustion. When she came to, the beaver noticed a group of fish jumping from the water, so she gathered all of her energy and waddled downstream. She climbed up a tree leaning over the creek-side and one by one, she grabbed the fish from the muddy waters. She reached out with her small fingers and tied each fish to the vines hanging down. Eventually all of the fish were caught and all died. Why did she do this? The beaver had perceived the fish as trying to escape the river and so she tried to "save" them. The fish, however, were not trying to escape at all. Instead, they were feeding on insects just above the water's surface (Haring, Titus, Stevens, & Estrada, 2012).

This story teaches an important lesson about diversity that can be applied to EAP practices within sovereign lands. What we perceive to be proper etiquette in EAP practices with one population may be meaningless or even harmful to another population, despite our best intentions and training. Differences in styles of thinking and cross-cultural communication give rise to potential concerns regarding the use of conventional EAP assessment, intervention, and referral techniques that are normed for EAP practice with mainstream organization, workplaces, and the communities in which they situate. Some key factors to be cognizant of include knowledge of occurrences of the past that influence sovereign Indigenous landscapes. These include occurrence of the past that influence current workplace health and community structures (historical trauma), awareness of the variance of Indigenous environmental context and their relationships with health care in the workplace setting, the importance of confidentiality, and the use of communication style between and among Indigenous groups.

Te Whakatōhea are a Māori iwi (tribe) located in the eastern Bay of Plenty region of New Zealand that has approximately 12,000 tribal members. The iwi is traditionally centered in the area around the town of Opotiki. The traditional territorial lands extend eastwards from Ohiwa Harbour to Opape along the coastline, and inland to Matawai. These lands have long held an abundance of food resources, particularly seafood, and most of the settlements are located near the coast. Whakatōhea's history of *Raupatu* (confiscation) from the early 1800s culminated in a series of events involving the loss of *mana* (power and control), the loss of leaders, the destruction of social structures which had a devastating impact on Whakatōhea identity, culture, economy, health, and well-being.

In recent years, the Whakatōhea Maori Trust Board (2010) embarked on a series of initiatives to support the transformation of Whakatōhea into a unified, purposeful nation that is independent and interdependent with other free and independent nations (p. 3). The foundation for this transformation has been the Ara Mai Whakatōhea Strategic Plan 2009–2013 (Whakatōhea Maori Trust Board, 2009) that informed a unique survey, He Oranga o te rohe o te Whakatōhea Wellbeing Survey 2010 (Whakatōhea Maori Trust Board, 2010), which is the only comprehensive iwi health survey undertaken in New Zealand to date. The survey involved face-to-face interviews with 750 registered adult members of Whakatōhea living in the Opotiki District and yielded a rich array of data on demographics, housing, general well-being, service utilization, health, social environment, and education (APR Consultants, 2010). The Whakatōhea Wellbeing Survey provides a reference point for the state of Te Whakatōhea health and well-being, an understanding of Te Whakatōhea aspirations for health and well-being, and has informed the development of economic, education, environmental, social, health, and cultural plans. This phase of tribal development is about radical transformation:

> how we see ourselves as whanau, hapu and iwi, how we influence and determine the fulfilment of our potential, how we express our uniqueness and creativity, and how we influence the design of the systems we live in, health, education, economy and environment. (Dickie Farrar, CEO Whakatōhea Maori Trust Board, April 15, 2010, personal communication)

The tribal values that underpin this direction are *Rangatiratanga* (acting with dignity and humility, taking ownership, expecting excellence), *Whanaungatanga* (relationship building), *Matawhanui* (we see the big picture), *Manaaki ki te tangata* (people matter), *Kaitiakitanga* (guardianship).

The Whakatōhea Maori Trust Board is the largest employer in Opotiki with approximately 100 staff across its commercial, education, health, and social services. One specific initiative that contributes to the transformation of services is the adoption of the Mauri Ora training program to provide staff with a framework focused on *kaupapa* Maori (Indigenous) principles and models and assist them to develop and implement solutions and strategies alongside *whanau, hapu*, and iwi that enable positive transformative outcomes (Te Korowai Aroha o Aotearoa, n.d.). The training equips *akonga* (students) with a solid philosophical base and foundation that validates the unique Maori belief systems, values, and practices; introduces them to the Maori conceptual framework for the prevention of family violence; and provides *kaupapa* Maori methods, tools, and practices to assist them when working to develop transformative outcomes. The Mauri Ora program supports the transformation of behavior by applying cultural constructs from Te Ao Maori (Maori worldviews) and taking into account environmental and contextual interference and influences from Te Ao Hurihuri (contemporary worldviews). Cultural constructs that are applied as practice tools within the program include:

- *Whakapapa*: collectivity and collective consciousness
- *Tikanga*: collective practice, cultural protocols
- *Wairua*: self-realization
- *Tapu*: self-esteem
- *Mauri*: inner values: influence and identity
- *Mana*: outer values: power and influence
- *Te Reo*: our identity.

Professional development and staff training has always been a priority, but the Mauri Ora program has broadened the focus beyond the technical skills into areas of cultural competency. Training our social service staff in the Mauri Ora program has had a number of direct benefits. It has allowed them to reconceptualize and reconfigure the services they provide to align more closely with the cultural values of the community. It has provided a greater focus on family and connectivity between the staff and clients as members of the same community, and it has allowed the staff to reflect on well-being within the workplace. The adoption of the Mauri Ora training has created opportunities for staff to consider the questions "How do we treat each other?" and "How do we support each other?"

Similarly the adoption of Results Based Accountability (RBA) as a framework for reporting has led to increased engagement and wellbeing amongst the staff. RBA is a means to manage service provision across the purchaser–provider divide, to ensure the efficiency and effectiveness of government spending, and to increase accountability and transparency of public and community sector organizations (Keever, Treleaven, Sykes, & Darcy, 2012). Management at the Whakatōhea Maori Trust Board has noticed changes in employee interactions since the introduction of RBA reporting and the Mauri Ora training and hypothesize that creating space to acknowledge and reinforce the positive action of staff, as well as affirm the positive outcomes within the community, can be directly linked to an increase in energy and commitment from the staff as well as higher levels of self-management and well-being.

The spillover benefits for the organization arising from integration of Indigenous models and outcome-based reporting has led to enhanced cultural competency (access to language training, use of cultural protocols in dispute resolution processes) and improved employee well-being (adoption of cultural strategies/models, recognition of positive staff contributions to community, energy, commitment and self-management).

Kanaka Maoli, more commonly known as Native Hawaiians, are the Indigenous Peoples of Hawai'i. Hawai'i's Indigenous People suffer some of the worst health disparities and socioeconomic status compared to other populations residing in the State. Native Hawaiians live 13 years fewer than those with greatest life expectancy (Park, Braun, Horiuchi, Tottori, & Onaka, 2009) and have a high infant mortality rate, which is more than twice that of White (7.9 vs. 3.5 per 1,000 live births) (Hirai, Hayes, Taualii, Singh, & Fuddy, 2013; Taualii, Quenga, Samoa, Samanani, & Dover, 2011). Significant contributors to the infant mortality disparity are education, age, and smoking; all of which could be improved with education and support services. Cardiovascular disease mortality is double, and diabetes-related mortality is 3 times higher than Whites (Mau, Sinclair, Saito, Baumhofer, & Kaholokula, 2009).

In an effort to address the disparities faced by Native Hawaiians and other Indigenous Peoples, the University of Hawai'i, Office of Public Health Studies, has recently launched a specialization in Native Hawaiian and Indigenous Health within the master of public health (MPH) degree. The need for such a program was identified by existing MPH students who felt the application of public health tools to serve the Native Hawaiian and Indigenous community did not meet its full potential. The need of the students was magnified by the need of the community to develop a highly skilled work force to serve and address the health needs of the community. This specialization was designed to prepare students with public heath skills and training necessary to serve Indigenous People globally and assist in addressing their health and wellness needs by contextualizing health determinants within historical and political frameworks. In addition, the specialization provides extensive training in culturally sensitive research ethics which is critical for safely and effectively implementing public health research and programs aimed to address and eliminate the inequities faced by Indigenous People (Burnette, Sanders, Butcher, & Salois, 2011; Usher, 2010).

HISTORICAL TRAUMA

Historical trauma is a traumatic or stressful era in history that alters the perceptions or behavior of a population, culture, or society. For Indigenous groups in North America, the most widely recognized historical trauma comes from the era of the boarding school. In the early 20th century, boarding schools were established to assimilate Native and First Nations peoples into mainstream culture. Indigenous children were removed from their homes, communities, and families and sent to institutions—sometimes very far away. The goal of the boarding schools was to "remove the Indian" and to replace their traditional way of life with that of the dominating society. Children were not allowed to speak Indigenous languages or practice ancient traditions. They were forced to speak foreign languages, become Christian or other religions of the era, cut their hair, and wear the clothing of other societies. Choosing not to follow the rules often resulted in severe abuse or death (Godlaski, Johnson, & Haring, 2006).

Because of this historical trauma, employees of Indigenous workforces may be hesitant to accept EAP practice by outside EAP professionals. This hesitation may not be due to the EAP professional's assessment, intervention, or practice methodology. Rather, the reluctance to participate in the EAP process may be due to influences, experiences, and perceptions passed down through generations. Boarding schools and other historical traumas within the Indigenous landscape left a generation of care givers that may have taught conflicting parenting styles. These learned styles of parenting may have reflected the abusive relationships that were projected onto them in boarding schools or their battle for cultural survival. As such, inappropriate social learning through modeling of their boarding school years might have produced atypical leadership styles and workplace behaviors.

In contemporary EAP practice, these residual effects of boarding schools and related trauma may form a barrier that creates mistrust between an EAP professional, the Indigenous employee, and family. Employees may see the EA professional as an expansion of mainstream governments. EAP professionals must be aware of these possible concerns, assess for them, and take them into consideration when practicing within the Indigenous workforce.

ENVIRONMENT

Key to working with Indigenous employees, families, and communities is knowledge of environmental differences, sovereign rights, and customs of the lands. Each tribe or band has its own unique environmental context, and there is a vast array of community colonization patterns, languages, and traditional practices. Outside EAP providers, affiliates, and organizations should keep a creative mind of awareness how to respectfully work in these unique sovereign landscapes. For instance, an EAP professional in the East working with the Seneca tribe in New York faces entirely different environmental contexts and cues than one in the North working with the Cree of Saskatchewan, Canada, or a Maori iwi of New Zealand. Work–life relationships differ from tribe to tribe and country to country. There are also differences from urban, rural, suburban, to reservation settings. An awareness of potential differences or similarities is essential.

It is also important to understand the movement of employees between family and community structures. For example, a Hopi employee might have a mother who lives on the reservation and a Navajo father who lives and works in the city, whereas the father's family resides on a neighboring Navajo reservation. The employee may spend the summers with his father's family, visit his mother in the city, and work in Navajo Country with his relatives. Such a lifestyle of family visiting is fairly commonplace for Indigenous employees and is not a sign of disrespect to EAP session dedication. From an Indigenous perspective, this is a way of communal being and family togetherness. Nonetheless, it can make scheduling and consistency of EAP challenging. In some cases, it may be beneficial for outside EAP professionals to have referral resources available in all of the employee's communities and be prepared to work with family members over a large regional landscape—possibly across international borders and in neighboring cities (Haring, 2009, 2011).

CONFIDENTIALITY

The ethic of confidentiality in Indigenous communities should be understood and applied in a nuanced manner. In a Māori context the ethic of confidentiality is always be balanced against an ethic of relationship and support (Hudson, 2004). The responsibility for community members to support each other can only be actioned within a space that allows for responsible disclosure. Due to the sensitivity of the issue some aspects of EAP practice will require a greater attention to confidentiality, however its application should be considered in the context of prevailing Indigenous values and protocols.

Confidentiality is essential to EAP practice. However, it is mandatory in small communities, and this is especially true for work within sovereign Indigenous lands associated with EAP contractual service areas. Indigenous communities and associated workplaces are often composed of smaller communities or family networks. These areas may not be found on any map, yet they have distinct names in the Indigenous landscape. In addition, many people on the reservation are related, whether by extended relations, unions, or through a number of social and community networks. As such, confidentiality is paramount. EAP professionals who do not promote strict confidentiality beyond that of Employee Assistance Professionals Association, Employee Assistance Trade Association, or other international standards risk long-term failure. As noted by Bernard Huber, Licensed Clinical Social Worker (personal communication, April 8, 2004), a long-time EAP practitioner in Indigenous landscapes, "Confidentiality in these close-knit communities is not only a strong ethical practice; it's the reputation of the profession and reflective of the organization that provides EAP services."

COMMUNICATION STYLES

The communication style of Indigenous employees may be different from that of mainstream workplaces and organizations. In fact, differences in styles of thinking and communication give rise to concerns regarding the use of conventional EAP assessment techniques within diverse cultures (Godlaski et al., 2006). Therefore, understanding communication styles, rapport building, and respectful turn-taking-style conversations may be beneficial skills for EAP professionals when providing services within Indigenous communities.

Communication styles should not be generalized from one Indigenous workplace and culture to another, but there are likely a few common elements. One is the use of silence. Indigenous employees often use "quietness" as a way to feel out the EAP professional, the EAP organization, or the process of EAP itself. It is often the case the employee is "reverse assessing" the EA professional to determine if they are willing to work with the practitioner. This is not a form of disrespect or disinterest. Rather, it is a means of communication and a form of nonverbal "reverse assessment" (Godlaski et al., 2006; Johnson et al., 2008). These authors also share that a second important communication practice is humor, laughter, and storytelling through joking. In work with Indigenous employees and family members, humor can be an important tool for building rapport. Humor is part of the healing process and may serve a number of roles for team building in the workplace. However, careful use of humor in EAP technique should be used in caution. This includes the use of culturally appropriate jokes, humor, and response. Conversely, the EAP professional should also be aware that the employee may be using the art of joking as a means to throw the EA professional off course from important topics that may arise during assessment.

It is also to be noted that relational communication frames interactions, and agenda based discussions with Indigenous communities are important and that cultural dissonance can emerge within Indigenous communities. Cultural dissonance can emerge in the workplace through a gendered or ethnic mismatch (Holland, 2009). Hook, Waaka, and Raumati (2007) contended that Māori can become disenchanted when mainstream workplaces does not support Māori employee development through recognition of important principles and connections such as *whanaungatanga* (relationship/togetherness/collectivity), *mana* (control), *mahakitanga* (humility), and *Wairuatanga* (spirituality). Cultural protocols that encourage the affirming of connections reduce cultural dissonance and can provide a process to balance the immediate importance and challenge of EAP discussions with supporting harmonious intergenerational relationships within the community.

MOLDING EAP FOR WORK WITH SOVEREIGN NATIONS

EAP practice is a circle of learning, application, and respect. Outside EAP professionals must remain open minded and promote their work within the Indigenous landscape in respectful and meaningful ways. Outside EAP professionals must also strive to develop respectful referral organizations and practitioners in multiple communities in which employees situate. Outside EAP professionals must also be open to self-evaluation of their place as a helper in the Indigenous community they serve by continually monitoring overall personal and organizational efforts and successes. Overall, EAP within Indigenous landscapes should be seen as a process of keeping an open mind, learning, trust building, and honoring workplace culture.

CONCLUSION

The art of EAP practice in Indigenous workforces is not a strict individual psychological direction but an array of psychology, social interaction, and community. Healing practices in Indigenous workforces present a contextual understanding of the holistic nature of human functioning that is unique to EA practice as opposed to many other helping professions, which tend to adopt a more individual-centered perspective to healing.

Further, it is the combinational use of principles represented in narrative accounts including the sharing of food, the disciplined use of self in a relationship with an individual or group, the group process and the efforts of groups upon individuals and the reciprocal influence of the individual upon the group and reciprocal influences of man and his total environment human, social, economic, and cultural—that provided data to support that historically Indigenous people promoted ideologies and concepts of wellness during various forms of assistance in and around duties associated with job function. These concepts found in an Indigenous framework include purpose, occurring under the conscious guidance of knowledge and values, which is patterned to some extent by methods that provides support to Indigenous healing practice.

Contracting with firms familiar with the nuances of working within the Indigenous landscape of sovereign nations is one means of addressing the complexities that may arise. These include such factors as counseling differences, understanding policy and regulatory differences, to community involvement and acceptance. Working with Indigenous-owned firms that hold a strong blend of Indigenous and varying cultural counseling staff, administrative help, and a well-rounded team also promotes Indigenous to Indigenous capacity building and increases the goal set forth in many sovereign Nations—the strive for self-determination through economic sovereignty.

EAP companies should also consider the incorporation of Indigenous philosophy and theory in the contracting process. This is represented by incorporating "good-minded EAP contracts" that are developed between the EAP firm and the sovereign Indigenous communities involved. The EAP contract has the ability to promote collaboration within a framework of mutual trust and cooperation. The contract will result in shared collaboration, mutual understanding, and will ensure that EAP work proceeds in a manner that is culturally sensitive, relevant, and beneficial to the workforce and communities.

Meaningful contracts also encourage and promote respect for each other. Respect is generated by understanding each other's social and cultural structures. The EAP organization and the Indigenous community cannot assume that they believe in the same things or share the same goals and expectations. Ongoing cultural sensitivity training for the EAP team and community awareness presentations will help develop a mutual understanding of the EA process for utilization. The concepts of "good-minded contracting" and honoring bidirectional respectful relationships are foundations learned from the Akwesasne Mohawk Nation and are cited from their protocol for the review of scientific research proposals on territories of the Seneca Nation of Indians (2011) that utilized these powerful guidelines with permission from the Akwesasne Task Force on Environmental Research and their Advisory Committee (1996).

SUMMARY

In today's growing Indigenous societies EAP is important. EAP when conducted properly and respectfully has the ability to improve workplace health and community health directed by the sovereign ability of the government through their workplace. EAP in Indigenous communities provides a unique means that is often less stigmatic than on-reserve or on-reservation health centers, for the provisions of a large range for employee wellness. Indigenous nations have the capability of ensuring the health of people through their workforce. Indigenous governments have the ability to guide EAP contracting that improves community health in respectful ways, yet staying within the boundaries of scientific EAP intervention principles. Finally, sovereign

Indigenous nations have the right and duty to promote the health of future generations in the community through the Indigenous workforce.

REFERENCES

Akwesasne Task Force on the Environment (ATFE) Research Advisory Committee (RAC). (1996). *Protocol for Review of Environmental and Scientific Research Proposals*. Retrieved from https://sites.google.com/site/atfeonline/documents

APR Consultants. (2010). *Whakatōhea Wellbeing Survey 2010 quantitative results summary report*. Ōpōtiki, New Zealand: Whakatōhea Maori Trust Board.

Brieland, D. (1977). Historical overview and special issue on conceptual frameworks. *Social Work, 22*(5), 341–346.

Burnette, C. E., Sanders, S., Butcher, H. K., & Salois, E. M. (2011). Illuminating the lived experiences of research with indigenous communities. *Journal of Ethnic & Cultural Diversity in Social Work, 20*(4), 275–296.

Chandler, M. J., & Lalonde, C. (1998). Cultural continuity as a hedge against suicide in Canada's First Nations. *Transcultural Psychiatry, 35*(2), 191–219. Retrieved from http://web.uvic.ca/~lalonde/manuscripts/1998Trans Cultural.pdf

Freeman, B. (2004). *Resiliency of a people: A Haudenosaunee concept of helping* (Unpublished master's thesis). McMaster University, Hamilton, Canada.

Godlaski, T. M., Johnson, J., & Haring, R. C. (2006). Reflections on ethical issues in research with aboriginal peoples. In J. Kleinig & S. Einstein (Eds.), *Ethical challenges for intervening in drug use: Policy, research and treatment issues* (pp. 281–306). Huntsville, TX: The Office of International Criminal Justice (OICJ), Sam Houston State University, Criminal Justice Center.

Government of Canada. (1996). *Report of the Royal Commission on Aboriginal People (RCAP)*. Ottawa, Canada: Author.

Haring, R. C. (2009). Private practice and the Native American client. *National Association of Social Workers, Private Practice Newsletter, Section Connection* (1), 9–10.

Haring, R. C. (2011). *EAP Practice with Native American Employees*. Employee Assistance Report. Impact Publications, Inc.: Waupaca, WI. 14(4), 1–3.

Haring, R., Titus, J., Stevens, L., & Estrada, B. (2012). Increasing the knowledge base: Utilizing the GAIN in culturally sensitive landscapes. *Fourth World Journal, 11*(2), 79–94.

Health Canada. (2003). *Statistical profile on the health of First Nations in Canada in Year 2000*. Ottawa, Canada: Government of Canada.

Hirai, A. H., Hayes, D. K., Taualii, M. M., Singh, G. K., & Fuddy, L. J. (2013). Excess infant mortality among Native Hawaiians: Identifying determinants for preventive action. *American Journal of Public Health, 103*(11), e88–95. doi:10.2105/AJPH.2013.301294.

Holland, C. (2009). *Workplace mentoring: A literature review*. Developed by Work and Education Research & Development Services Supported by the Industry Training Federation. Retrieved from https://akoaotearoa.ac.nz/download/ng/file/group-4/n3682-workplace-mentoring—a-literature-review.pdf

Hook, G., Waaka, T., & Raumati, P. (2007). Mentoring Māori within a Pakeha framework. *MAI Review, 3*(1), 1–3.

Hudson, M. (2004). *He Matatika Maori: Maori and ethical review in health research* (Unpublished master's thesis). Auckland University of Technology, Auckland, New Zealand.

Jamerson, J. F. (1909). *Narratives of New Netherland, 1609–1664.* New York, NY: Charles Scribners Sons.

Johnson, J., Baldwin, J., Haring, R. C., Wiechelt, S. A., Roth, S., Gryczynski, J., & Lozano, H. (2008). Essential information for disaster management and trauma specialists working with American Indians. In A. Marsella, J. Johnson, P. Watson, & J. Gryczynski (Eds.), *Ethnocultural perspectives on disaster and trauma: Foundations, issues, and applications* (pp. 73–113). New York, NY: Springer SBM Publishing.

Keever, L., Treleaven, L., Sykes, C., & Darcy, M. (2012). Made to measure: Taming practices with results based accountability. *Organisation Studies, 33*(1), 97–120.

Mau, M. K., Sinclair, K., Saito, E. P., Baumhofer, K. N., & Kaholokula, J. K. (2009). Cardiometabolic health disparities in Native Hawaiians and other Pacific Islanders. *Epidemiologic Reviews, 31*, 113–129.

MacMillan, H. L., MacMillan, A. B., Offord, D. R., & Dingle, J. L. (1996). Aboriginal health. *Canadian Medical Association Journal, 155*(11), 1569–1578.

McIntosh, J. (1844). *The origin of the North American Indians: With a faithful description of their manners and customs, both civil and military, their religions, languages, dress, and ornaments: to which is prefixed a brief view of the creation of the world . . . concluding with a copious selection of Indian speeches, the antiquities of America, the civilization of the Mexicans, and some final observations on the origin of the Indians.* New York, NY: Nafis & Cornish. Retrieved from http://digital.library.wisc.edu/1711.dl/History.McIntosh

The National Congress of American Indians. (2006). *Methamphetamine in Indian Country: An American problem uniquely affecting Indian Country.* Retrieved from http://www.justice.gov/archive/tribal/docs/fv_tjs/session_1/session1_presentations/Meth_Overview.pdf

Office of Applied Studies, Substance Abuse and Mental Health Services Administration. (2005). *Methamphetamine use, abuse, and dependence: 2002, 2003, and 2004. The National Survey on Drug Use and Health Report (NSDUH).* Rockville, MD: Author.

Olson, L. M., & Wahab, S. (2006). American Indians and suicide: A neglected area of research. *Trauma, Violence & Abuse, 7*(1), 19–33.

Park, C. B., Braun, K. L., Horiuchi, B. Y., Tottori, C., & Onaka, A. T. (2009). Longevity disparities in multiethnic Hawaii: An analysis of 2000 life tables. *Public Health Reports, 124*(4), 579–584.

Parker, A. C. (1913). *The code of Handsome Lake, the Seneca prophet.* Education Department bulletin/University of the State of New York State Museum; 163. Albany, NY: University of the State of New York.

Public Law 103–50, 103rd Congress Joint Resolution 19, Nov. 23, 1993.

Seneca Nation of Indians. (2011). *Protocol for review of scientific research proposals on Territories of the Seneca Nation of Indians.* Retrieved from http://www.sni.org

Shewell, H. (2004). *'Enough to keep them alive': Indian welfare in Canada, 1873–1965.* Toronto, Canada: University of Toronto Press.

Strickland, C. J., Walsh, E., & Cooper, M. (2006). Healing fractured families: Parents' and elders' perspectives on the impact of colonization and youth suicide prevention in a Pacific Northwest American Indian Tribe. *Journal of Transcultural Nursing, 17*(1), 5–12.

Taualii, M. M., Quenga, J. A., Samoa, R. A., Samanani, S., & Dover, D. (2011). Liberating data: Accessing Native Hawaiian and other Pacific Islander data from national data sets. *AAPI NEXUS, 9*(1), 1–7.

Te Korowai Aroha o Aotearoa. (n.d.). Retrieved from http://www.tekorowai.org

Usher, K. (2010). Indigenous higher degree research students making a difference to the Indigenous health agenda. *Contemporary Nurse: A Journal for the Australian Nursing Profession, 37*(1), 102–106.

Whakatōhea Maori Trust Board. (2009). *Ara Mai Whakatōhea strategic plan.* Ōpōtiki, New Zealand: Author

Whakatōhea Maori Trust Board. (2010). *He Oranga o te rohe o te Whakatōhea Wellbeing Survey.* Ōpōtiki, New Zealand: Author

White Bear, J. (2003). *National Aboriginal youth participation and evaluation report.* Ottawa, Canada: National Aboriginal Health Organization.

Employee Assistance Programs in Australia: Evaluating Success

ROBERT-LEIGH COMPTON, BBus, MEcon, LittD

Newcastle Business School, University of Newcastle, Newcastle, Australia

JOHN G. MCMANUS, BA, MA, PhD

Mind & Matter Consulting, North Sydney, Australia

Employee Assistance Programs (EAPs) are a vital aspect of organizational support and a significant and important element of Human Resources Management. The efficacy of an EAP will therefore have strong implications for the effective functioning of the people processes within an organization. It is incumbent upon organizations to assess the success of their program, its effectiveness, and its efficiency. An employer survey was conducted with 44 organizations that currently provide EAPs to their employees. The study was conducted in 2010, 2011, and 2012 and was based on a range of organizations with a total of approximately 50,500 employees who are in receipt of EAP services, from providers who are members of the Employee Assistance Professional Association of Australasia. The results concluded that EAPs do indeed attend to a wide range of psychological issues and that organizations benefit widely from the existence of EAPs. Furthermore, the study revealed that a close connection between EAPs and Human Resources Management is shown to be beneficial in terms of the broader organizational issues. Even though there is evidence of extensive satisfaction with EAP services it is also evident that there is opportunity to improve the level of monitoring and evaluation of such services to ensure their part in adding value to the organization.

INTRODUCTION

Much of Human Resources Management (HRM) literature will emphasize that an organizations' employees are its most valuable asset (Kramar, Bartram, Gerhart, Hollenbeck, & Noe, 2014; Nankervis, Compton, Baird, & Coffey, 2011; Stone, 2011). The literature claims that successful organizations tend to be those that are committed to aiding their employees to manage and deal with a range of issues and problems they may face (Buon & Compton, 1990). Yet it is interesting to note that the issue of counselling of employees and assessing their overall well-being is not so well understood or evaluated and would benefit from more research attention (Alker & McHugh, 2000; Csiernik, 2004).

The provision of Employee Assistance Programs (EAPs) for employees and their direct family members as a feature of HRM processes has gathered greater prominence in recent years (Arthur, 2000; Berridge, 1999; Kirk & Brown, 2003, 2005; Kirk-Brown & Wallace 2004; Wolters Kluwer, 2004). The provision of EAPs to organizations is usually instigated by the Human Resources Division or managers assigned to people processes within the organization.

It is assumed that the appointment of professional assistance by way of an EAP provides for an effective management of emotion as it affects the workplace. EAPs consist of a range of services centered around counselling support that are designed to assist individuals in the work context, promote individual health, and diminish the chances of negative impact of personal or work problems on the work environment and ultimately on the profitability and viability of organizations. An examination of the available literature in the field of HRM shows that EAPs as a topic is a relatively small subject area in proportion to the available literature on other HR initiatives such as performance management, training, remuneration (Compton, 2006; Csiernik, 2004).

The motivation to establish employee counselling through an EAP is essentially that there is recognition at the organizational level that the emotional lives of people at work and at home at times causes considerable stress and strain and ultimately affects work performance. Early intervention is seen as vital as is top management support for the program (Kaplan & Dietz, 2007). In addition, a change in culture is also essential where the organization recognizes a mind-set that acknowledges the health and wellness issues of the whole person. Work–life strategies must be available to all employees and their families across the entire organization (Jones & Paul, 2011), as people seek to manage the demands of their various life domains.

There has always been a question about the efficacy and value of EAP interventions and programs. There has been growing perception amongst many large organizations that the provision of EAP services to their employees has many direct and indirect advantages and that the direct advantages include reduced costs in terms of sick leave, absenteeism, and workers compensation (McManus, 2008). The indirect advantages include improved morale and an improved reputation for the organization. Empirical evidence relating to EAPs has emerged from research in various parts of the world. Berridge and Cooper (1994) in a U.K. study reported that "payoffs of EAPs can be very positive across a range of objective performance criteria" (p. 4). King (1994) in another U.K. study reported that sickness absence events and days lost to sickness decreased significantly as a result of EAP activity. In the United States, McShulskis (1996) found that EAPs improved morale and productivity and decreased absenteeism and lowered overall healthcare costs. In another U.S. study, Wirt (1998) stated, "EAPs reduce absenteeism, healthcare costs and disciplinary action" (p. 158).

In other organizations, EAPs have evolved from a strategy of employee wellness to one that also includes a risk management component. Early intervention can clearly help to avoid problems such as substance abuse, mental illness, lost time accidents, and reduced absences. A proactive EAP can also assist in avoiding the cost of litigation (Kaplan & Dietz, 2007).

To some, EAPs can represent a "big brother" meddling in employees' private lives. To others, they are yet another management fad and a waste of time. A more positive approach is adopted by current day EAP providers that see an EAP as an effective strategy for assisting employees when personal or work-related problems are affecting their work life, family life, social life, and work–life harmony. The programs are characterized by effective, early, and minimum intervention. They offer a wide range of strategies and aim at resolving many varied problems (Compton 1988; McManus, 2008).

There is perhaps a distinctive flavor to Australian EAPs derived from the history and local circumstances. Kirk and Brown (2008) referred to "a somewhat unique service-delivery model, grounded in local legislative and industrial influences" (p. 353). They also made the point that counselling is the core activity of Australian EAPs but that there are EAP providers endeavoring to offer a wider range of services, integrated services, such as work–life and wellness programs, that seek to be useful and strategic for the organization and efficacious for the individual in receipt of such professional services. They suggested, however, that there is an enduring shortfall of understanding of EAPs in the Australian context: "there remains among the human resource community a wide-spread lack of understanding of the role of EAPs, and of their strategic integration within a firm's human resource practices" (p. 362).

The promotion and development of services and programs requires a robust and effective relationship between HR professionals and EAP professionals. To this end strong regular and open communication is essential between HRM and EAP professionals. It requires ongoing evaluation of the effectiveness of EAPs and effective strategies to ensure that employees are fully aware of the availability of their programs. In these circumstances it is argued that there are distinct benefits for individuals in receipt of services and for the organization as a whole.

METHOD

The sample for this survey involved six EAP providers across Australia each members of the Employee Assistance Professional Association of Australasia (2010), the Australasian peak body in the EAP field. The six EAP providers who participated provide counselling services to 44 organizations with a total of 50,500 employees. The sample involved responses from small businesses (14%), medium-sized businesses (50%), and large businesses (36%). Each major industry type was selected including banking and finance, construction and engineering, education, entertainment, public sector, health care, hospitality and tourism, insurance, information technology, manufacturing, media, mining, telecommunications, and transport. A 15-item questionnaire was administered by phone after prior agreement with the organization's HR representative or other manager who had responsibility for the conduct of the EAP program. The selection was based on the advice of the providers as to which organizations were willing to participate in the study. Any selection bias (Rossi & Freeman, 1993) was minimized by the broad range of participant organizations. Any uncertainty or ambiguities were clarified during the course of the interview. The questionnaire is a semistructured research tool with a number of open-ended questions included in the final question in regard to the value and evaluation of EAPs. The questionnaire was designed by the authors.

The survey is the largest ever conducted in Australia and has a dual focus:

1. To consider the nature and usefulness of EAP counseling in Australian organizations.
2. To determine the appropriateness and extent of evaluation of EAP counseling.

Although the first question has been subject to a number of surveys over the past ten years (Compton, 2006; Compton & McManus, 2010; Kirk & Brown 2003, 2005). there has never been a serious attempt to review the perceived value of EAPs the ways that organizations evaluate the worth and value to organizations across a variety of industry settings. This survey has been successful in providing answers to both research questions.

RESULTS

The survey results consider specific answers in relation to set questions as well as open-ended responses to the invitation to provide comments

TABLE 1 Why Did Your Organization Introduce an Employee Assistance Program?

Reason	Percentage
Align business strategy with organizational Human Resources strategy	6
Component of an integrated Human Resources strategy	9
To implement best practice	15
Personal problems affecting productivity	4
Help retain key staff	4
Boost employee engagement	9
Support for employee health and well-being	18
Reduce risk of litigation	5
Perceived duty of care	12
Stress management tool	8
Other	10

regarding EAPs overall and the issue of evaluation. The following results highlight the central issues dealt with in the survey.

The results indicated that the reasons that organizations have for the introduction of an EAP are many and varied (see Table 1). However the three most important reasons are support for employee health and well-being, 18%; to implement best practice, 15%; and perceived duty of care, 12%. Only 6% of respondents saw that effective counselling provided a link between business strategy and HRM strategy.

The survey found that the linkages of EAPs to business processes were also varied (see Table 2) but that many respondents, 42%, considered that EAPs were an important part of their occupational health, safety, and wellness initiatives. Surprisingly only a small number, 8%, considered that EAPs were important within their strategies aimed at absence management. Of specific note is that only 6% and 4% saw a link between counselling and performance review and career planning respectively. Counselling was linked to discipline and grievance procedures in 15% of the responses indicating that these organizations perceived that counselling was in integral part of these processes. Indeed, counselling is quite a separate process and must

TABLE 2 Is Your Employee Assistance Program Linked with Any of the Following Business Processes in Your Organization?

Option	Percentage
Performance review	6
Career management	4
Absence management	8
Education and development	10
Occupational health, safety and wellness inactive(s)	42
Discipline and grievance procedures	15
Attraction and retention strategy	8
Other	4
None	3

TABLE 3 What is Your Organizations' Employee Assistance Program Utilization Rate (Actual or Estimated)?

Option	Percentage
No relevant records	24
0%–2%	10
2.1%–4%	24
4.1%–6%	16
6.1%–8%	7
Above 8%	19

never be confused with disciplining. The focus is very different. Counselling is developmental. Disciplining is punitive in its very nature.

The range of utilization rates reported by respondents was large (see Table 3). Only 23% reported that their EAPs were operating in the normal expected rate for a healthy EAP (McManus, 2008) of between 4.1% and 8%. Ten percent reported particularly low levels of utilization of between 0% and 2%, and 19% reported quite high levels of above 8%. Most surprisingly, 24% of respondents reported that they kept no relevant records. Of interest here is that an EAP (or any other HRM program) cannot be evaluated if accurate records are not maintained.

The occupational categories for employees using the EAPs was found to be quite wide spread, including a small percentage for family members, 5% (see Table 4), but the majority of respondents, 51%, reported that there were no relevant records, which again is of concern when HRM is under pressure to show that their programs add value.

The survey found that there was a wide age distribution of employees using the EAPs (see Table 5) with the highest percentage, 14%, belonging to the age 40 to 49 years group. It is of interest that 10% of respondents were in the age group 50 to 59 years. Anecdotal evidenced gained in the follow up interviews indicate that the major concern for this age group is, perhaps not surprisingly, superannuation concerns and preparation for retirement. Once

TABLE 4 Percentage of Those Employees Using the Employee Assistance Program

Option	Percentage
No relevant records	51
Executives or senior managers	2
Middle managers, including supervisory	6
Non-management professionals	11
Skilled trade or technical	9
Clerical or sales	7
Unskilled laboring or general duties	9
From families of your employees	5

TABLE 5 What Are the Ages of Employees Who Have Used Your Employee Assistance Program? Include Family Clients if Known. Please Indicate Using Percentages (Actual or Estimated)

Option	Percentage
No relevant records	52
Younger than age 20 years	1
20–29 years	10
30–39 years	12
40–49 years	14
50–59 years	10
60 + years	1

again, the majority of respondents, 52%, reported that there were no relevant records.

The issues that presented most commonly to the EAP (see Table 6) were personal relationships or family problems 31% and work related stress, 15%. There were 24% of respondents who reported that there were no relevant records. Despite widespread media concern, harassment and bullying at work accounted for only 2% of cases presented.

The perceived benefits of EAPs to organizations (see Table 7) largely centered on workplace relationships with the three main benefits being improved employee relations, 20%; improved morale, 17%; and less stress in the workplace, 13%. Interestingly the bottom line financial issues were rated much lower in the range of responses with increased productivity, 8%, and increased bottom line/profitability, 4%, being seen as quite inconsequential by the sample of respondents.

In a surprising result for the researchers 58% of respondents replied, in response to the question, "Have you established and used a method for

TABLE 6 What Percentage (Actual or Estimated) of Employees Have Presented to Your Employee Assistance Program with the Following Issues?

Option	Percentage
No relevant records	24
Personal relationship or family problems	31
Work related stress	15
Emotional disturbances	10
Financial pressures	5
Other[a]	15

[a]Other includes:.

Workplace interpersonal conflict 4%.

Alcohol or substance abuse 2%.

Harassment and bullying at work 2%.

Retirement or pre-retirement issues 1%.

Other nonspecified 6%.

TABLE 7 Have You Demonstrated That Your Employee Assistance Program Has Provided Any of the Following Benefits?

Option	Percentage
Reduced absenteeism	9
Reduced turnover	7
Improved morale	17
Improved employee relations	20
Increased productivity	8
Increased engagement	8
Increased bottom line/profitability	4
Less stress in the workplace generally	13
Other	3
None	11

TABLE 8 In What Ways Have You Measured the Effectiveness of Your Employee Assistance Program?

Option	Percentage
Employee Assistance Program provider	11
Impact on work	6
Employee feedback	31
Surveys	22
Take up rate	8
Independent assessment	6
Other	17

evaluating the effectiveness of the EAP?" that they had no method of evaluation. However the remaining 42% of respondents replied that they did regularly evaluate their EAP and used a variety of methods to establish the level of effectiveness (see Table 8). The two main methods that were reported were direct employee feedback, 31%, and the use of surveys, 22%.

OPEN-ENDED QUESTIONS

In response to the question, "Please provide any other comments you may have regarding EAPs and their evaluation?" (see Table 9), there were a range of responses ranging from affirming comments about the value of EAPs to admissions of inability in relation to evaluation of their EAP. Some respondents directed their comments to providers and asked for direct help in the development of improved ongoing methods of evaluation.

One respondent described EAPs as "an invaluable part of our employee engagement and well-being programs." Another respondent commented that EAPs are "a benefit to the employee and a protection for the manager." A further comment was that "EAPs are an essential tool." One respondent who felt that the task of evaluation was indeed a difficult one stated

TABLE 9 Please Provide Any Other Comments You May Have Regarding EAPs and Their Evaluation

Comment	Responses
- I am sorry however most data is old and unreliable. Next year!	8
- Would like a recommendation of a common way of evaluating our service providers.	10

- Our provider provided exceptional:
   - service
   - intervention
   - outcomes
   - education
	14

- Invaluable part of our employee engagement & wellbeing programs.	15
- A simple template should be supplied to access & use within the business to measure the effectiveness of the EAP	18
- Keen to have a better relationship with the provider—should tailor services to the needs of the company	
- Would like the capacity to buy on products—for example, due to the high access rate for pre-existing mental illness, we would like to be able to purchase awareness sessions to train managers to better respond to these employees	
- Greater flexibility of use, provider is only available 2 days a week	
- Management support for the EAP concept is useful for the benefit of the employee + protection for the manager	21
- Essential good practice	22
- Recommendations as to how to evaluate would be welcome	23
- We have worked very hard as an organization to have EAP services viewed as an essential tool in workforce and career development and management. I believe we have broken down the stigma sometimes associated with seeking counseling and, as such, staff are accessing the service and consider they are getting better results from it. It has also helped that there has been continuous improvement in the quality of services offered by EAP providers.	24
- Please tell us how to do this! This is an area whose EAP providers could take more initiative in conclusion surveys of employees who use their services.	28
- Very hard to ascribe any of the benefits (of EAPs) listed in Q14 to an EAP alone	
- We treat our EAP service confidential. It is between the client and EAP services.	29
- We have reviewed the cost of EAP but overall are happy with the service	38
- Evaluating EAP is a tricky area. Often the EAP is a small part of a larger Human Resource strategy to improve workplace culture & staff satisfaction. I feel it is important for staff to be able to access an external support program	40

"evaluating EAP is a tricky area. Often the EAP is a small part of a larger HR strategy." The requests for assistance were strongly expressed, "Please tell us how to do this!" and "this is an area where EAP providers could take more initiative." Yet another respondent stated, "a simple template should be supplied to access and use within the business to measure the effectiveness of the EAP."

Another surprising finding clearly shown in the tables is the number of organizations that do not keep records that would assist them to evaluate their EAPs.

DISCUSSION

This study considered the question of whether EAPs are a valued aspect of organizational support and a significant and important element of HRM. The research considered how organizations that implement EAPs review the effectiveness and efficiency of the programs, whether they conduct evaluations and if so how they conduct these assessments. The findings suggest that EAPs attend to a wide range of psychological issues that involve workplace issues and personal issues. The results reveal that there is a close connection between EAPs and HRM and that EAPs are perceived as beneficial to the organization. It was however concluded that despite a high level of satisfaction with EAP services that the monitoring and evaluation of these services could be greatly improved.

The research was a qualitative study and the findings suggest that EAPs are put in place primarily due to a need to support employee health and well-being. In addition the programs are seen to address a perceived duty of care and a desire to implement best practice in the area. Overall EAPs are viewed as an important part of an organization's occupational health, safety and wellness initiatives.

The study's findings can clearly be seen to address the research questions of effectiveness of EAPs and evaluation of such programs. The discussion that follows pays particular attention to these central research questions.

The range of utilization reported in the study was quite variable, but the authors noted that a high percentage of respondents (34%) reported that their programs had notably low rates of utilization of 0% to 4%. Azzone et al. (2009) suggested that higher rates of utilization require a strong ongoing campaign of promotion and regular worksite activities.

The occupational groupings were widely spread with a lower participation rate existing for executives or senior managers. This may suggest a reticence on behalf of senior managers to engage with EAP professionals based on a concern that they may be subject to criticism about the nature of the workplace and in particular workplace stress. Nobrega, Champagne, Azaroff, Shetty, and Punnett (2010) reported that respondents in their study consistently encountered barriers when seeking access to management. Such barriers and ongoing attitudes potentially decrease opportunities for dialogue that may lead to program improvements but also perhaps decrease the likelihood of senior managers making use of such programs when they, personally, are in need.

The EAPs were found to be in receipt of a wide range of presenting issues including both personal issues and work related issues. Dallimore and Mickel (2006) referred to the importance of EAPs in providing support to employees and their families and as a method of promoting quality of life. The main issues presenting to the EAPs considered in this study were personal relationship or family problems. This finding is consistent with previous studies who have found that relationship issues and family pressures are regular presenting issues to such programs (McManus, 2008).

The benefits of EAPs to organizations from the perspective of HR managers or other equivalent managers, who have responsibility for the conduct of the EAP in their organization, is that the main benefits are improved employee relations, improved morale, and a reduction in stress in the workplace. Other advantages such as reduced sick leave, reduced workers compensations, and reduced absenteeism (McManus, 2008) seem to be either viewed as of lesser importance or alternatively are simply not being monitored or studied. There was evidence of an awareness of the importance of workplace stress as an issue for some of the managers in this study. Nobrega et al. (2010) commented that "substantial barriers exist for EAPs to engage employers in primary prevention related to workplace stress" (p. 293), but the study results suggest that there is an opportunity to further develop communication between HR professionals and EAP professionals and in so doing improve the chances of achieving progress on this issue and a wide range of workplace issues.

A central part of this research was the issue of how organizations actually evaluate their programs and determine effectiveness. The majority of respondents (58%) in this sample stated that they had not established and used a method of evaluation. The remainder of the sample (42%) reported that they had relied upon employee feedback and surveys as well as provider information and comments to determine the success or otherwise of their program.

A number of themes were determined in relation to the open-ended reponses. The themes included statements that EAPs are essentially part of a larger HR strategy and that there is a high level of satisfaction with the programs. It is seen as "essential good practice," but overwhelmingly there is evidence of insufficient or inadequate means of evaluations. Furthermore the results reveal an emphatic request for assistance to make effective evaluations of such services.

It is perhaps appropriate to consider the reasons that Australian organizations have for the engagement of EAPs. Kirk (2005) demonstrated that there are distinctly different reasons for adoption of a program as compared to the reasons for the continuance of EAPs for organizations. Adoption is often based on "adverse workplace conditions or events beyond the usual range of the oganisations's coping mechanisms" (p. 91). In other words, organizations are likely to have felt internal pressure in response to change issues or they have been attempting to respond to trauma or critical incident management. In contrast reasons for continuation of a program shift to humanistic rationales, "humanistic concerns emerge as later rationalisations for the continuance of the program" (p. 91).

The issue of evaluation remains central to this study. Yamatani, Sanangelo, Maue, and Health (1999) in an analysis and evaluation of a university EAP stated that it is essential that the organization, engaging such services, specify their EAP polices, the major goals of the program and to set objectives. In this way, it is argued, it is then possible to measure goals and objectives that are consistent with polices and agreements and allow for a systematic evaluation. Yamatani et al. stated that major goals of evaluation were to "generate information pertaining to the program's service adequacy, program effectiveness, client satisfaction, costefficiency and cost-saving" (p. 107). Yet the respondents in this study demonstrated little interest in establishing a structured method of evaluation, let alone a "systematic evaluation."

Shakespeare-Finch and Scully (2005) used qualitative and quantitative methods to evaluate an EAP for a particular Australian ambulance service. They comment on the paucity of literature and research on the topic and that much of the evaluation that does take place is reliant upon the more superficial aspects such as usage rates and broad descriptive detail. In contrast during their study they thoroughly considered the component parts of the EAP and the specific satisfaction of employees with those components. The overall results revealed a positive picture of the effectiveness and success of the EAP: "results demonstrate that the services provided are frequently accessed, attract high levels of staff satisfaction and that the higher levels of satisfaction were demonstrated to occur regardless of age, gender, length of service, work role or work region" (p. 89).

The importance of evaluation was emphasized by Masi (1997) when she referred to the dual requirements of attaining appropriate professional support for employees and their family members as well as providing value for money invested in the program by the organization "to evaluate whether the company's investment in the EAP is actually helping its employees. It is an employer's responsibility to ensure the effectiveness of the program and to determine if change is required" (p. 378). Masi (1997) also made the point that a regular process of evaluation by an organization allows for that organization to consider if the program is reflecting the philosophy of the company, operating in a way that is consistent with the agreement, cost effective, meeting clinical needs and improving employees' levels of functioning. Masi (2011) highlighted the need for EAPs, in their own right, to combine a business model with a professional model to meet a broad range of objectives and improve the practices of EAPs, allowing for "a professional practice group that successfully combines a for profit business with a professional practice model" (p. 1). Such cooperation would clearly be of benefit to all parties.

The results of this study would seem to suggest that the monitoring and evaluation of EAPs in Australia is at best patchy or perhaps even insufficient and inadequate. The responsibility would seem to lie with the organization, in particular the HRM function, as well as the provider of such services, that is, the EAP providers. Although the results suggest that EAPs are viewed as important and successful programs, there is a need for greater cooperation to conduct systematic evaluations on a regular basis so that the best clinical, organizational and economic outcome can be achieved. The possibility of improvement and development in the EAP field requires the fostering of even closer and more extensive ties between EAPs and HR Management.

REFERENCES

Alker, L. P., & McHugh, D. (2000). Human resource maintenance? Organisational rationales for the introduction of employee assistance programmes. *Journal of Managerial Psychology, 15*(4), 303–333.

Arthur, A. R. (2000). Employee assistance programmes: The emperor's new clothes of stress management? *British Journal of Guidance & Counselling, 28*(4), 549–559.

Azzone, V., McCann, B., Levy Merrick, E., Hiatt, D., Hodgkin, D., & Horgan, C. (2009). Workplace stress, organizational facts and EAP utilization. *Journal of Workplace Behavioral Health, 24*(3), 344–356.

Berridge, J. (1999). Employee assistance programs and stress counselling: At a crossroads? In C. Feltham (Ed.), *Controversies in Psychotherapy and Counselling* (pp. 252–268). London, UK: Sage.

Berridge, J. R., & Cooper, C. L. (1994). The employee assistance programme: Its role in organizational coping and excellence. *Personnel Review, 23*(7), 4–20.

Buon, T., & Compton, R. L. (1990). Alcohol and other drug programs in the Australian workplace. *Business Insights, 36*(6), 24–29.

Compton, R., & McManus, J. (2010, September). Workplace counselling. Is it the business of business? *Management Today,* 26–28.

Compton, R. L. (1988). *Employee Assistance Programs – A case of concerned management or big brother?* (Working Paper No. 40). Sydney, Australia: School of Business, Nepean College of Advanced Education.

Compton, R. L. (2006). Workplace counselling down under: Caring HRM or a license to print money? *Business and Informatics – Current Trends; College of Social Sciences Warsaw, Book of Readings,* 1496–1503.

Csiernik, R. (2004). A review of EAP evaluation in the 1990s. *Employee Assistance Quarterly, 19*(4), 21–37.

Dallimore, E., & Mickel, A. (2006). Quality of life: Obstacles, advice, and employer assistance. *Human Relations, 59*(1), 61–103.

Employee Assistance Professional Association of Australasia. (2010). *What is an employee assistance program?* Retrieved from http://www.eapaa.org.au

Jones, E., & Paul, R. (2011). How Employee Assistance Programs can build a culture of health. *Behavioural Healthcare, 31*(6), 32–36.

Kaplan, D., & Dietz, P. (2007). Use employee assistance to manage risk. *Occupational Health and Safety, 76*(7), 82–94.

King, S. (1994). Counselling through employee assistance programs. *Management Development Review, 7*(2), 38–40.

Kirk, A. (2005). Employee assistance program adoption in Australia: Strategic management or 'knee-jerk' solutions? *Journal of Workplace Behavioral Health, 21*(1), 79–95.

Kirk, A., & Brown, D. F. (2008). Chapter 18: Australian perspectives on the organizational integration of employee assistance services. *Journal of Workplace Behavioral Health, 20*(3–4), 351–366.

Kirk, A. K., & Brown, D. F. (2003). Employee assistance programs: A review of the management of stress and well being through workplace counselling and consulting. *Australian Psychologist, 38*(2), 138–143.

Kirk, A. K., & Brown, D. F. (2005). Australian perspectives on the organizational integration of employee assistance services. *Journal of Workplace Behavioral Health, 20*(3/4), 351–366.

Kirk-Brown, A., & Wallace, D. (2004). Predicting burnout and job satisfaction in workplace counselors: The influence of role stressors, job challenge and organizational knowledge. *Journal of Employment Counseling, 41*(1), 29–37.

Kramar, R., Bartram, T. K., Gerhart, B., Hollenbeck, J. R., & Noe, R. (2014). *Human resource management: Strategy, people, performance* (5th ed.). Sydney, Australia: McGraw.

Masi, D. A. (1997). Evaluating Employee Assistance Programs. *Research on Social Work Practice, 7*(3), 378–390.

Masi, D. A. (2011). Redefining the EAP field. *Journal of Workplace Behavioral Health, 26*(1), 1–9.

McManus, J. G. (2008). *A Kleinian analysis of organisations: Implications for employee* health and well-being (Unpublished doctoral dissertation). Business School University of Queensland, Queensland, Australia.

McShulskis, E. (1996, May). Employee Assistance Programs effective, but underused? *HR Magazine, 21*, 19–20.

Nankervis, A., Compton, R. L., Baird, M., & Coffey, J. (2011). *Human resource management: Strategies and processes* (7th ed.). South Melbourne, Australia: Cengage.

Nobrega, S., Champagne, N. J., Azaroff, L. S., Shetty, K., & Punnett, L. (2010). Barriers to workplace stress interventions in employee assistance practice: EAP perspectives. *Journal of Workplace Behavioral Health, 25*(4), 282–295.

Rossi, P. H., & Freeman, H. E. (1993). *Evaluation: A systematic approach* (5th ed.). Newbury Park, CA.

Shakespeare-Finch, J., & Scully, P. (2005). A multi-method evaluation of an Australian emergency service Employee Assistance Program. *Employee Assistance Quarterly, 19*(4), 71–91.

Stone, R. (2011). *Human resource management* (7th ed.). Milton, UK: Wiley.

Yamatani, H., Sanangelo, L. K., Maue, C., & Health, M C. (1999). A Comparative analysis and evaluation of a university Employee Assistance Program. *Employee Assistance Quarterly, 15*(1), 107–118.

Wirt, G. L. (1998, November). The ABCs of EAPs. *HR Focus, 12*, 158.

Wolters Kluwer (UK) Limited. (2004). *UK: The benefits of Employee Assistance Programs*. Sydney, Australia: CCH Australia Limited.

Using an Interactive Self-Assessment Tool to Strengthen Your Employee Assistance Service

LILIANA DIAS, MA, PhD candidate

Faculty of Psychology and Educational Sciences, University of Leuven, Leuven, Belgium

AUDREY EERTMANS, PhD, INGE VAN DEN BRANDE, PhD, YASMIN HANDAJA, MA, and SOFIE TAEYMANS, MA

ISW Limits, Leuven, Belgium

DEBORA VANSTEENWEGEN, PhD

Faculty of Psychology and Educational Sciences, University of Leuven, Leuven, Belgium

ISAT was developed by ISW Limits, a spin-off of the University of Leuven (Belgium). It stands for Interactive Self-Assessment Tool, which is an online screening about well-being at work. ISAT provides employees with individual feedback about their mental health and well-being at work. In addition, the tool provides tailored self-management advice as well as information about how and where to get support from the employer and the Employee Assistance Program provider. To the employers, ISAT offers group results in order to help companies target interventions.

Interactive Self-Assessment Tool (ISAT) is based on a previously validated questionnaire, the Short Inventory on Stress and Well-Being (S-ISW; Vander Elst, Eertmans, Taeymans, De Witte, & De Cuyper, 2011) and was further complemented by a questionnaire about coping styles. The tool is thus composed of three tests (i.e., well-being indicators, perception of the work situation, and coping styles), broken down in several scales. After completing a test the respondent receives immediate feedback including graphs with the

---

Color versions of one or more of the figures in the article can be found online at www.tandfonline.com/wjwb.

person's score compared to a large multisector benchmark as well as tailored personal advice with regard to coping-strategies and when necessary, referral to internal or external mental health services (including Employee Assistance Program [EAP]). The tool also contains the possibility of sharing the results with a counselor or team leader. The objective of the tool is prevention and early intervention for stress and motivational issues, building resilience at the workplace by stimulating self-management at the individual level, and enabling early stage interventions at the group level within the company.

ISAT is aligned with the main goal of the EAP field to improve productivity and healthy functioning at the workplace, particularly by providing direct and confidential advice and psycho-educational support, by using constructive confrontation and motivation to address problems that affect job performance, and by actively promoting EAP services when available.

The tool has been implemented in different organizational settings and several markets (e.g., Belgium, The Netherlands, France, Japan, United States of America). Results will be presented about the uptake, usefulness, evaluation, and outcome of the tool for employees, for companies, and for employee assistance providers. A randomized controlled study also evaluated the added value of presenting immediate tailored feedback by measuring its impact on proactive behavior of employees. Special attention will be given to the advantages of using the tool in combination with employee assistance services.

INTRODUCTION

Well-being at work is a concept increasingly attracting attention from researchers and the private sector. ISW Limits, a spin-off company of the University of Leuven (KULeuven, Belgium), has recently developed and globally commercialized an innovative web-based tool, denominated ISAT, with the main goal of providing insight into employee's well-being and reducing psychosocial risks at the workplace that may have an impact upon well-being.

ISAT was designed to help organizations implement the entire psychosocial risk management process, following the general principles within the European Framework Agreement on work-related stress (2004), and the recommended dynamic risk management system (i.e., screening, evaluation, actions, information). ISAT is a tool for "screening," which also provides support in terms of action planning and offers a structure for informing employees and orientating them toward the existing support within their company.

According to the Belgian legal framework, employers have a legal obligation to conduct a global prevention policy or a well-being policy, managers are expected to enact the policy, and employees at all levels should participate in and contribute to the well-being policy of the company. When the required internal expertise is insufficient, organizations should call upon external expertise provided by external services for prevention and protection at work or consultancy firms.

ISAT DEVELOPMENT

ISAT is an online self-assessment tool, which returns immediate individual feedback to the employee as well as personal advice about individual stress and motivation levels and how to cope with problem situations. To the employer, the tool offers results at group level (e.g., department, site, divisions, teams, functions) as well as insights in the main factors that impact on stress and motivation.

Theoretically, the tool is based on the comprehensive and evidence based model for well-being at work developed by ISW Limits in 2007 (see Fig. 1). This model refers to major indicators of well-being at work (e.g., global job satisfaction, pride of one's job and company, versus stress signals and undesirable behaviors at work). ISAT includes measurements of physical, mental, and social health perception of the employees at work, hereby tapping into the core dimensions of the World Health Organization's (1946) definition of health as "a state of physical, mental and social well-being." Further, the model describes different levels of intervention (i.e., primary, secondary, and tertiary) and takes into account different layers of the work situation on which one might intervene (i.e., person, task, team, leadership, organization, and policy), while acknowledging the influence of the socioeconomic context external to the company. As such, it aids to analyze the risk

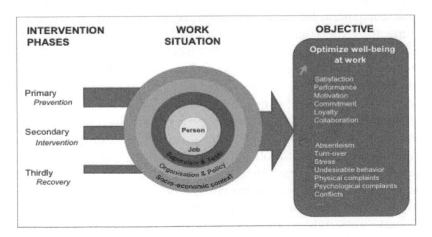

FIGURE 1 Inventory on Stress and Well-Being Limits Intervention Model. © 2007 ISW Limits. Reproduced by permission of ISW Limits. Permission to reuse must be obtained from the rightsholder.

factors and to determine leverages for promoting well-being and motivation at work and for preventing or managing stress.

This model is in line with the rich tradition of theoretical models for stress and well-being at work, pointing at different factors that might play a role in well-being at work such as motivation, autonomy, job characteristics, effort-reward balance, job demands, social support, and job resources (Bakker, Demerouti, de Boer, & Schaufeli, 2003; Demerouti, Bakker, Nachreiner, & Schaufeli, 2001; Hackman & Oldham, 1976, 1980; Herzberg, 1966; Karasek, 1979; Karasek & Theorell, 1990; Siegrist, 1996).

Herzberg's (1966) two-factor theory suggests that there exist two independent sets of circumstances that drive employee satisfaction and motivation, namely, hygiene factors and motivator factors. Hygiene factors (named dissatisfiers), if absent, are postulated to make employees unsatisfied at work, motivator factors (named satisfiers) are postulated to make employees feel good about their jobs.

The job characteristics model proposed by Hackman and Oldham (1976, 1980) explains individual responses to jobs (e.g., job satisfaction, sickness absenteeism, personal turnover) as a function of job characteristics, moderated by individual characteristics (Roberts & Glick, 1981). The model defines the core job characteristics as skill variety (i.e., breadth of skills used at work), task significance (i.e., opportunity to complete an entire piece of work), feedback (i.e., amount of information provided about effectiveness of job performance), and autonomy (i.e., degree to which the job provides substantial freedom, independence, and discretion in determining goal-directed behavior at work).

The demand-control model (DCM; Karasek, 1979; Karasek & Theorell, 1990) hypothesizes that strain will be highest in jobs characterized by the combination of high job demands and low job control—"high-strain jobs." In contrast, task enjoyment, learning, and personal growth will be highest in jobs characterized by the combination of high job demands and high control—"active learning jobs," Even faced with intensively demanding jobs, employees with greater decision latitude are expected to use all available skills, enabling conversion of aroused energy into action through effective problem solving.

The effort-reward imbalance model (ERI; Siegrist, 1996) emphasizes the reward, rather than the control structure of work. The ERI model assumes that job stress is the result of an imbalance between effort (i.e., extrinsic job demands and intrinsic motivation to meet these demands) and reward (i.e., in terms of salary; esteem reward and security/career opportunities, such as promotion prospects, status consistency, and job security). The core assumption is that a lack of reciprocity between effort and reward will lead to arousal and stress, which may, in turn, increase cardiovascular risks and other stress reactions.

The job demands-resources (JD-R) model (Bakker, Demerouti, de Boer, et al., 2003; Demerouti et al., 2001) defends that job demands precede burnout, whereas job resources determine engagement. The model proposes a dual pathway to employee well-being. Job demands are the most important predictors of such outcomes as exhaustion, psychosomatic health complaints, and repetitive strain injury (RSI) (e.g., Bakker, Demerouti, & Schaufeli, 2003; Hakanen, Bakker, & Schaufeli, 2006). Job resources are generally strong predictors of work enjoyment, motivation, and engagement (Bakker, Hakanen, Demerouti, & Xanthopoulou, 2007; Bakker, van Veldhoven, & Xanthopoulou 2010).

Building on these theoretical models and on its vision model, ISW Limits developed a questionnaire to analyze the working conditions and shed a light on the most important factors that impact on stress and well-being at the workplace: the Short Inventory on Stress and Well-being (S-ISW). For instance, the S-ISW includes items that measure either burnout (i.e., exhaustion, cynism—the contrast of "enthusiasm" on ISAT, and reduced professional efficacy—labeled as "decreased feeling of competence" in ISAT; Maslach & Leiter, 1997; Maslach, Schaufeli, & Leiter, 2001) or engagement (e.g., pride in one's job, job centrality; Bakker & Demerouti, 2008; Schaufeli & Bakker, 2003).

The main aim in developing the S-ISW questionnaire was to create an efficient tool, which would provide a broad view of work-related characteristics and psychosocial outcomes, highlighting positive and negative characteristics of the work situation, while minimizing completion time, be clearly and simply formulated so that all employees, regardless of their education level, would be able to fill out the questionnaire.

The S-ISW had been validated (see also further) and used for several years by ISW Limits in paper and online surveys, when it was integrated in the new ISAT as its core questionnaire.

ISAT STRUCTURE

The first part of ISAT consists of a set of demographic questions such as gender, age group and level of education, and general questions about the user's professional context (e.g., staff category, seniority within his company, contract type, and direct and indirect supervision responsibilities within the company). Based on the answers to these preliminary questions, the reference group is defined to which the participant will be compared in the self-assessments.

After this, participants are guided through three tests (i.e., Well-being at Work, Work Situation, Coping), which cover nine dimensions or self-assessments. All along the tests, and for each dimension, participants receive immediate feedback and advice related to their score and its position toward their reference group, as you can see in the Figure 2.

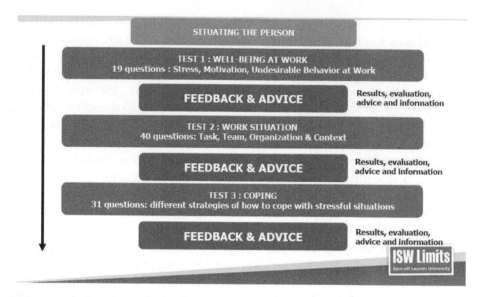

FIGURE 2 Interactive Self-Assessment Tool structure. © 2009 ISW Limits nv. Reproduced by permission of ISW Limits. Permission to reuse must be obtained from the rightsholder.

The first test consists of three indicators of well-being (S-ISW): stress complaints (eight items), motivation (seven items), and undesirable behavior at work (four items).

Stress complaints include indicators of lack of occupational well-being and health, which can be considered various types of symptoms: emotional (e.g., mood complaints, tension, irritation), cognitive (e.g., feelings of insufficiency, distraction, and concentration problems) or physical (e.g., sleeping problems, fatigue, neck of back aches and headaches, exhaustion, and persistence strain). Examples of items for this dimension are: "I generally feel unhappy or depressed" and "I am distracted or find it hard to concentrate on my work."

Motivation covers positive emotional, motivational and behavioral well-being indicators, as well as attitudes toward the job and the company, such as enthusiasm in the job, job satisfaction, job centrality and performance, functional loyalty, pride in one's job, and pride in one's company. A few examples of items for this dimension are "I work less enthusiastically than in the past," I'm generally satisfied with my job," and "I'm proud of my job."

Undesirable behavior at work refers to harassment or mobbing, but also to other kinds of undesirable behavior in the workplace such as sexual harassment and violence. "In my company, people do harass each other at times (more than innocent teasing)" and "At times I feel I am victim of other undesirable behavior (discrimination, violence and aggression, sexual harassment, etc.)" are examples of the items for this dimension.

The second test of ISAT focuses on five different dimensions or layers within the work situation: job demands (12 items), task motivators (seven items), team (four items), organization (13 items), and context (four items).

Job demands refers to psychological demands of work such as travel time, work–life balance, workload, flexibility granted by employer, overtime, work complexity, emotional demands, the possibility to take breaks, impact of mistakes, physical demands, difficult outsiders, and demanding responsibility.

Examples of items that measure job demands: "I can easily combine my job with my private life," "I feel that I have to work too hard," and "My job is physically demanding."

Task motivators include aspects of work that make work attractive or challenging, such as autonomy, training, responsibility, skill utilization, personal development, task variation, and understimulation. Examples of items for this scale: "My job implies great responsibilities," "I can personally grow in the job I perform," and "There is enough variety in my job."

Team items describe team characteristics such as social atmosphere, support from colleagues, support from one's supervisor, and feedback from the supervisor. "The atmosphere in my department/division is pleasant," "I can count on my colleagues' support," and "My immediate supervisor gives me feedback about the way I do my work" are examples of items of this dimension.

Organization describes characteristics, policies, and practices of the company that strongly influence perceptions of organizational support and well-being at work such as materials, remuneration, staffing, participation, values, work organization, information, physical conditions and safety, clear expectations, policy, staff attraction, staff retention, and knowing a confidant within the company.

Examples of organization items are "I can do my job safely and hygienically," "I know exactly what others expect from me at work," and "I have confidence in the policy of my company."

Socioeconomic context includes items that refer to the potential influences from the external social or economic context of the company, on employees' perceptions of occupational stress and motivation, such as job insecurity, perspectives, position on job market and fear of changes. "I worry about my job's future," "I see a bright future for myself in the company I am working for," and "There are sufficient opportunities on the job market for people like me" are examples of items that assess influences from the socioeconomic context.

The third and final test assesses coping styles of respondents, such as problem solving, getting control over one's thoughts, social support, emotional expression, waiting and avoiding, depressive reactions, palliative reactions like drinking, active entertainment/relaxation, and taking a break. Example of coping items are "I try to forget the problem," "I talk to someone about it," and "I keep physically active (sport, gardening)."

MULTILEVEL FEEDBACK AND ADVICE

ISAT provides different kinds of feedback to the individual users and to the company. To the individual users, it provides personalized feedback on their perceptions of stress and well-being at work, comparing them to their reference group (see also higher). ISAT reference and cut-off scores are based on a benchmark of S-ISW respondents from 65 companies extended with a random sample of 9,500 employees, resulting in a total sample of 31,899 employees.

Next to a personal score and comparison with a reference group, the employee also gets specific feedback that applies to the person's specific score. In the interface of the ISAT tests, this feedback is formulated as brief explanations, accompanied by links that will orientate the employee to more elaborate advice texts. These texts consist of general information on stress and work motivation, and information about different coping styles, or how to cope with stress and specific stressful situations, how to increase one's motivation and how to cope with specific risk factors in the work situation. A large part of their content were originally based on the syllabus of a stress management training, translated and validated by ISW Limits in collaboration with the Leuven University. Other information is based on the experience of the ISW Limits consultants within companies (Van Daele, Van Audenhove, Vansteenwegen, Hermans, & Van den Bergh, 2013).

The advice texts are located in the ISAT Library, which is accessible from each screen in the tool and which participants are free to explore, consult and print out. For a given company, the tool also refers to specific actors and partners (company doctor, HR, EAP), workshops and all other well-being initiatives within the company.

Note that it is here that the connection is made in ISAT between the results and the feedback that the employee is receiving on the one hand, and the services the EA provider is offering on the other hand. Employees in need for further support receive the possibility to directly access the telephone or online help provided by the EAP. For instance, a face-to-face session can be requested immediately through the EA-service system.

Finally, employees can receive, save, and print an individual feedback report and also share their results and feedback, via e-mail with their supervisor, the EA provider or any person of trust within or outside the company.

At the level of the company, group results are provided. External and internal benchmark analyses can be conducted. External benchmarking is performed by comparing group results to the ISW Limits database that has been adjusted to the profile of the company (i.e., a default weighting of the benchmark by sociodemographic profile, and if desired also by economic sector). Internal benchmarking is based on the comparison of groups within the company with the global picture of the company.

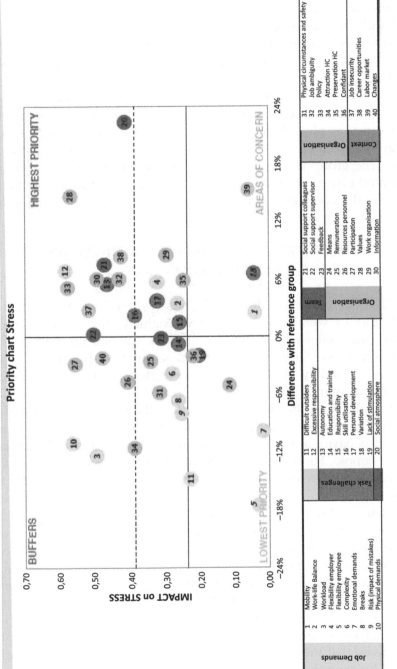

FIGURE 3 Example of impact analysis feedback for the company.

For specific groups within the company, such as business units, both these external and internal benchmarking are combined into a sort of Strengths, Weaknesses, Opportunities and Threats (SWOT) analysis, indicating specific strengths and weaknesses of the business unit compared to the external and internal reference group.

Next to this benchmarking, impact analyses are performed to reveal the risk factors within the work situation that have the strongest relation to stress and well-being within the company (see Fig. 3).

These analyses at group level eventually give an indication to the company of potential leverages for well-being at work and themes for its preventive action plan. Namely, either strengths or weaknesses that have an impact on well-being, and that hence can be considered buffers or priorities. The group report of the ISAT can help the company to establish goal-oriented actions to address risk factors, and also to monitor the evolution within the company of specific key indicators of well-being at work.

PSYCHOMETRIC EVALUATION OF INDICATORS OF WELL-BEING ON ISAT

Vander Elst et al. (2009) conducted a large-scale psychometric evaluation of the indicators of well-being within ISAT, namely, the Stress Complaints, Motivation and Undesirable Behaviour at Work scales from the S-ISW questionnaire (see above; Short Inventory on Stress and Well-being). In this study, validity and reliability analyses were conducted for two versions of the S-ISW, the Dutch and the French version.

The results of the factor analysis on the indicators of well-being showed that the proposed three-factor model, with stress complaints, motivation and undesirable behavior at work as dimensions, had a good fit with the data for the whole sample. Furthermore, the factor structure of the indicators of well-being revealed to be cross-culturally invariant, and convergent validity of the dimensions stress complaints and motivation with similar measures was verified.

Predictive validity was also investigated in this study, by looking at the association of stress complaints, motivation and undesirable behavior at work, with absence frequency, absence duration, and doctor visitation frequency one year later. Results showed that stress complaints were positively associated with doctor visitation frequency, motivation was negatively related to absence frequency due to illness and, finally, undesirable behavior at work was positively associated with absence duration.

An analysis of the test–retest reliability of the three dimensions of the S-ISW showed that the scores on stress complaints, motivation and undesirable behavior at work were very stable over a period of at least 10 days. Also, Cronbach's alpha coefficients for stress complaints, motivation, and undesirable behavior at work indicated adequate reliability (not lower than .80).

In conclusion, the findings of this study demonstrated the validity and the reliability of the indicators of well-being of the S-ISW, and hence of the specific test of ISAT that measures these indicators of well-being. Thus, this test of the ISAT can be considered a solid tool to conduct research to help companies in the developing of a well-being policy or prevention plan, and also to meet with statutory regulations.

As regards other tests of ISAT, work situation and coping, ISW Limits performs regular analyses of validity and reliability on its benchmark database. For the risk factors of the S-ISW, which are the scales included in the work situation test of ISAT, Cronbach's alpha have been found to vary between a high .85 and a lower .56 (for organization, respectively, context). Some of these indices are lower than those found for the well-being indicators of the S-ISW. This can be explained by the fact the scales have been compounded from a very diverse and interrelated range of work characteristics, mainly on the basis of a content criterion, namely, the "level of intervention" (task, team, organization, context). Stated differently, these scales should not be considered to be traditional "effect indicator" scales that are constructed around factor analysis and parallel items. Instead we consider the risk factors to be "cause indicators" designed around a formative logic that combines different things to form a broader construct (Bollen & Lennox, 1991). Still, the reliability indices are generally acceptable allowing to compute scale scores. Also, fairly strong cross-cultural stability in these figures has been observed between the Dutch and French versions of the S-ISW.

Concurrent validity of the S-ISW scales was demonstrated through regression analysis: measured in a cross- sectional design, the 40 risk factors were found to explain 49%, 68%, and 36% of unique variance (R^2) in, respectively, stress, motivation, and undesirable behavior. For the coping test of ISAT, reliability indices in a test sample of 2,000 participants, revealed Cronbach's alpha varying between .54 and .81 (i.e., wait/avoiding .73; problem solving .80; active entertainment/relaxation .68; social support .81; emotional expression, .70; getting control over thoughts .67; depressive reactions .75; taking rest .64; palliative reactions .54).

More recently (2012–2013), a validation study of ISAT was performed by ISW Limits for a Japanese-translated version of the instrument. The study concluded that the Japanese version of the ISAT tests have strong psychometric qualities in terms of reliability and validity. The results also strongly resembled the results found in the European validation study, in that similar Cronbach's alpha were found (stress: .85, motivation: .85, and undesirable behavior: .83). Concurrent validity was established, with the risk factors explaining 63% of the dimension stress complaints, 69% of the dimension motivation and 47% of the dimension undesirable behavior. Predictive validity was tested over a period of one year, with the risk factors measured during Wave 1 (2012), explaining 46%, 48%, and 40% of total variance in the well-being indicators (respectively, stress complaints, motivation, and undesirable behavior) measured during Wave 2 (2013).

THE EFFECT OF IMMEDIATE FEEDBACK: A CONTROLLED STUDY

ISAT uses personalized feedback as a way to promote behavioral change and proactive behavior. This personalized feedback is an important and unique characteristic of ISAT.

Research has shown that personalized feedback is effective in promoting behavior change, for instance, in alcohol use (Larimer & Cronce, 2007) and in drinking behavior by a web-based approach (Doumas & Andersen, 2009), in nutrition education (DiClemente, Marinilli, Singh, & Bellino, 2001), and in bulimia treatment (Schmidt et al., 2006). For e-mental health applications at the workplace however, such evidence is lacking.

In an experimental study, the immediate feedback delivered directly to the respondent was manipulated, and two different versions of ISAT were implemented within random groups of employees of several companies who were invited in the study through a snowball procedure. A total of 148 participants were randomly divided into an experimental condition ($n = 72$), which received feedback immediately after answering the self-assessment questionnaires, and a control condition ($n = 76$), which received delayed feedback. One month after their participation, a second measurement took place (n experimental condition $= 34$; n control condition $= 30$).

Overall satisfaction and the intention to actively solve problems were measured with the evaluation questionnaire previously developed and used by ISW Limits. Self-efficacy was measured using the Dutch adaptation of the General Self-Efficacy Scale (Schwarzer & Jerusalem, 1995). Proactive attitude was measured by the Proactive Attitude Scale (Schmitz & Schwartzer, 1999), and Empowerment by the Worker Empowerment Scale (Lesli, Holzhalb, & Holland, 1998).

The results show that employees who received immediate feedback are more willing to use the tool in the future and to discuss their situation with others compared to the control condition. No significant differences were found, for proactive attitude, self-efficacy and empowerment aggregated measurements.

ISAT WITHIN THE EAP FIELD

The use of ISAT as a self-assessment tool for employees within companies is strongly aligned with the main goal of the EAP intervention field, which is to improve productive and healthy functioning at the workplace. It accomplishes this by providing direct and confidential feedback, advice and psychoeducational support to employees, stimulating proactive behavior to openly discuss problems and start addressing issues that are affecting job performance. Also, by providing direct access to EAP resources available in their company. For EAP providers, ISAT can help to reinforce their services in different ways.

First, an ISAT customized to EAP's individual clients and companies will offer the clients direct specific advice, information, and feedback, as well as a different channel for referrals to EA counselors. Second, when individual ISAT users decide to share the report containing their individual results with a case manager and an EAP counselor, this gives the EAP a heads up: a preliminary insight into the employee's work situation and well-being that should otherwise be analyzed during an intake or a counseling session. In other words, ISAT may well allow counselors to faster target the issues faced by their individual client. On a collective level, this sharing of ISAT individual reports may help EAP's to find more efficiency on calls and counseling sessions.

Third, EAP providers can gain profound insight on how they can improve their support towards client companies in the development of their well-being policy based on the collective report with group results of ISAT.

Within an EAP core technology model (Roman & -Blum, 1985), ISAT can accomplish assessment, constructive confrontation with employees, and referral processes. When considering a more recent comprehensive EAP service model proposed by Kurzman (2013), ISAT also responds to a change in focus from management to the individual user in EAP: it establishes itself as a benefit and a new resource for all workers, not only on a tertiary level of intervention ("care"), but also on a primary and secondary level ("prevention").

Although management reports can still be created, indicating risk factors and groups at risk to develop action plans, the employee will benefit immediately from the individual feedback and advise. This can already be considered as a first preventive global action (primary prevention).

Also, employees who are at risk for (secondary prevention) or already suffering from (tertiary prevention) stress complaints, demotivation, burn-out, or undesirable behavior are selectively encouraged to get in touch with the EAP. Lowering the threshold for contacting the EAP will enhance tackling problems sooner, before they start escalating and become more cumbersome to solve. In other words, the effectiveness of the EAP is enhanced.

The possibility to share the individual report of the ISAT with the EAP professional (at the employee's request) can help the EAP professional to get a quick review of the employees' perception of the work situation when he or she gets in touch: the main issues and the positive sides of the situation are immediately visible. This information helps the EAP professional during the conversation. In other words, the ISAT enhances also the efficiency of the EAP.

IMPLEMENTATION AND EVALUATION OF ISAT IN DIFFERENT SETTINGS

ISAT was implemented at Company 1, one of the biggest players in Belgium in the communications sector. It was the first company that integrated ISAT in its larger psychosocial well-being program, in 2007. The company had a long history of offering EAP (individual therapy) and stress resilience trainings to its employees, which were very effective programs. At the same time though, there was a need for a tool that would integrate all the prevention services offered to the employees, and that would allow individual employees to assess their well-being and receive advice and support, and allow the company to get a group report based on these individual assessments. These were the reasons for this company to implement the ISAT. ISAT has been used in this company ever since for different reasons and at different levels (see also Fig. 4):

- As a stress audit tool (tool for psychosocial risk analysis) at the level of the whole company
- As an audit tool for specific teams at risk (e.g., high stress problems, problems of mobbing ...)
- As a tool for each individual employee who wants to assess his/her own well-being at work and want to know more about possible risk factors in his/her own specific work situation and how to deal with those problems/factors

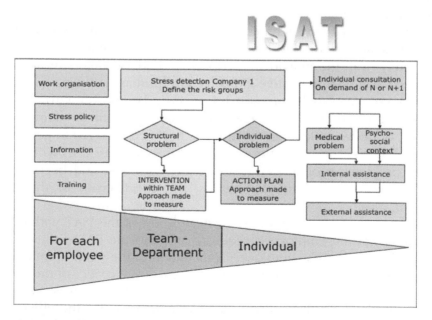

FIGURE 4 Different implementation goals with Interactive Self-Assessment Tool.

- As input and follow-up/evaluation tool for the individual counselling sessions (EAP)
- As input and follow-up/evaluation tool for the stress resilience trainings.

The ISAT in this company is coordinated by Corporate Prevention Protection, but other partners (e.g., the social unit, the training department, HR,etc.) are also involved.

Company specific information is added, such as programs, procedures, and values, training overviews, and referrals to internal and external support services. Together with the company, ISW Limits also developed a paper version of ISAT for employees who do not use a personal computer.

In 2008 ISAT was launched in the whole company. It was available through the intranet of the company. After one month, already 1661 (11% of the population) employees had used ISAT. Two hundred and nineteen employees also filled in the evaluation questionnaire which was added at the end of the tool, after the ISAT tests. Sixty-seven percent evaluated the tool as positive, 21% had a mixed opinion and 12% gave a negative evaluation.

Some quotes of the employees were "It's a very professional tool," "Very interesting and valuable," "Very clear and easily manageable," "The real power of the tool is of course the fact that you can immediately look into your results and compare with the norm group."

The average consultation and completion time of ISAT (i.e., reading of feedback included) was 42 minutes, and 86% spent less than an hour with ISAT. In terms of the individual report utilization, 26.6% of participants printed their results and 13.8% shared the results with someone else. The advisory texts in the Library section of ISAT were used by 67.6% of employees, more in particular, the pages about sharing results with your supervisor (28%), dealing with problems and stressors (28%) and causes of stress (27%) were consulted. 21% of the users clicked on the information about the Human Resources department, work–life, or other internal programs available within the company.

The general evaluation of the tool was very positive as shown in Figure 5, particularly about user friendliness of ISAT (83%), the fact that the tool is very complete (66%), the intention to recommend the tool to colleagues (62%), and the intention to use the tool in the future (63%).

With regard to the recommendations given, participants answered the question, "To what extent do you plan to apply the advice that you have received, to your work situation?" Thirty-five percent responded positively, and 49% of the participants evaluated that ISAT could be of value for them to improve their own well-being. Eighty-two percent of the employees stated that they would choose a more proactive problem-solving attitude toward problems in the future, 79% would use emotional coping towards finding a solution when facing issues (see Fig. 6).

General Assessment of the Tool

I would recommend this tool to my colleagues | 5% 9% 23% 45% 17%
I would use this tool in the future | 4% 9% 24% 46% 17%
I think the tool is generally too long | 8% 20% 25% 37% 10%
I think the tool is rather complete | 2% 9% 23% 53% 13%
I think the tool is very useful to me | 3% 11% 34% 39% 13%
The tool meets my expectations | 3% 10% 36% 41% 9%
I plan to discuss the results with someone | 22% 28% 30% 17% 4%
I think it's good that I can share with someone else my results | 8% 20% 34% 28% 9%
I find it interesting that I can choose what questionnaire or test | 1% 40% 24% 48% 23%
I think the tool is generally very user-friendly | 1% 5% 11% 56% 27%

Legend: Very Negative, Rather Negative, Neutral, Rather Positive, Very Positive

0% 10% 20% 30% 40% 50% 60% 70% 80% 90% 100%

FIGURE 5 Percentage of very positive, rather positive, neutral, rather negative, and very negative responses to 10 evaluation questions about the use of the tool.

Another organizational setting where ISAT was implemented was at a Belgian site of Company 2, a major international producer of fast-moving consumer goods. The ISAT was implemented as part of a larger program related to mental and physical health and well-being, and was coordinated on the site by the local health, safety & environment department (HSE). Company specific information was added, such as programs, procedures, and values, training overviews, and referrals to internal and external support services. Of the total number of employees of the site, 30% participated in the ISAT (457/1521). An evaluation study was conducted about five months after the launch of the tool, inviting all users up to that date to answer to a set of questions by means of a Likert-type five-point rating scale. The study focused on nature of use, general impression of the tool, evaluation of the

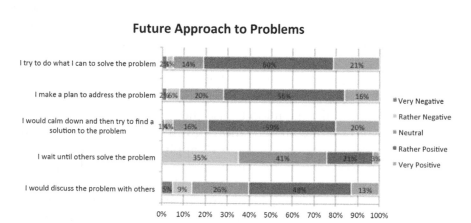

Future Approach to Problems

I try to do what I can to solve the problem | 2% 14% 60% 21%
I make a plan to address the problem | 2% 6% 20% 56% 16%
I would calm down and then try to find a solution to the problem | 1% 4% 16% 59% 20%
I wait until others solve the problem | 35% 41% 21% 3%
I would discuss the problem with others | 5% 9% 26% 48% 13%

Legend: Very Negative, Rather Negative, Neutral, Rather Positive, Very Positive

0% 10% 20% 30% 40% 50% 60% 70% 80% 90% 100%

FIGURE 6 Percentage of very positive, rather positive, neutral, rather negative, and very negative responses to six questions about attitudes toward problem solving.

questionnaires and graphical feedback, consulting and evaluation of advisory texts (Library), evaluation of the personal report and the option to share it with other person(s), and evaluation of the tool in general. Of all users, 37 employees (8%) completed the entire evaluation.

The average time of consultation and completion was 53 minutes, and the general evaluation was positive (21 of 37 employees gave a clearly positive evaluation in general terms). Participants evaluated the questions as clearly formulated (95% indicated a positive evaluation on the five-point rating scale), understandable (94%), and relevant (71%). The list of questions was not too long (80%). Participants evaluated the graphs as well designed (77%), easy to interpret (65%), understandable (80%) and recognizable (80%). 35.1% of the participants consulted the texts from the Library and considered the advice texts to be interesting (90%), relevant and meaningful (80%), and to be sufficiently focused on their personal situation (40%). 77.10% of the participants made use of the opportunity to receive their results in an individual report, considered the report useful (85%), and valued the possibility of sharing the results with someone (55%).

Feedback about the tool and its implementation in the company was also given by the HSE department: the tool, already in use since 2010, was considered an excellent framework for adding company specific information and orientate employees toward the existing support from internal departments and persons, and from external partners to the company.

In a second type of implementation, ISAT was offered more recently as a personal risk manager (PRM) to clients of another provider of mental health treatment programs in the Netherlands, Company 3. This organization integrated ISAT in its individual counselling series for persons with work-related problems. In this context, the therapist asks the client to fill out PRM at the start and at the end of the series of sessions. The therapist can consult the feedback reports of his or her client and can discuss it with the client and use it as input for the counselling/therapy.

One year after integrating the PRM as one of the online tools the therapists can use during their counselling, the PRM was evaluated by the therapists themselves. Eighty-five persons evaluated the PRM. A large majority of the respondents were aware of the tool (82.4%), and 60% of them use the tool for clients with work-related problems at the start of the trajectory. Only 25% uses the tool at the beginning and at the end of the trajectory. When questioned if there was a significant decrease in the client's PRM results overtime, 31% of participants said yes. Fifty percent discuss the results of the PRM during consultation with the client.

In general, about one third of the respondents considered PRM to be a useful tool with a clear added value for the client, because it gives a clear analysis of the work situation for each individual and helps the therapist understanding the issues faced by the individual at work.

CONCLUSION

We can conclude that ISAT is an evidence-based tool, which presents strong validity and reliability as an individual assessment tool within organizational settings. Some specific features of the tool, such as the immediate personalized feedback, receive good usability feedback from the users (e.g., overall satisfaction and intention to actively solve problems), but need further testing of their impact on proactive attitude towards problems at the workplace.

Within three organizational settings where ISAT was implemented and evaluated, the users' evaluation of the tool reveal a good uptake and on average a very positive evaluation of its usefulness when assessing work from a broad and complete psychological, physiological and social point of view. Although some consider the tool to be a little bit long, most of its users consider that questions, texts, images, and library links are well organized and easy to comprehend and follow. From the point of view of therapists who offer the tool to their clients for assessment and follow-up reassessments of well-being at work, one third of professionals considered the tool very useful for their client, as well as to themselves for reviewing goals and intervention plans.

ISAT has a strong value proposal to EA providers, their client companies, and individual users. It presents itself as an assessment tool that gives direct feedback, advice, and access to EAP information and services using an online platform available to all employees. Also, by collecting data about individuals' perceptions it enables companies to improve work design, and health policies. As such, it allows a move forward from the tertiary focus of traditional EAP core technology to more primary and secondary interventions.

REFERENCES

Bakker, A. B., & Demerouti, E. (2008). Towards a model of work engagement. *Career Development International, 13*(3), 209–223.

Bakker, A. B., Demerouti, E., de Boer, E., & Schaufeli, W. B. (2003). Job demands and job resources as predictors of absence duration and frequency. *Journal of Vocational Behavior, 62*(2), 341–356.

Bakker, A., Demerouti, E., & Schaufeli, W. (2003). Dual processes at work in a call centre: An application of the job demands–resources model. *European Journal of Work and Organizational Psychology, 12*(4), 393–417.

Bakker, A. B., Hakanen, J. J., Demerouti, E., & Xanthopoulou, D. (2007). Job resources boost work engagement, particularly when job demands are high. *Journal of Educational Psychology, 99*, 274–284.

Bakker, A. B., van Veldhoven, M., & Xanthopoulou, D. (2010). Beyond the demand-control model: Thriving on high job demands and resources. *Journal of Personnel Psychology, 9*(1), 3–16.

Bollen, K. A., & Lennox, R. D. (1991). Conventional wisdom on measurement: A structural equations perspective. *Psychological Bulletin, 110*(2), 305–314.

Demerouti, E., Bakker, A. B., Nachreiner, F., & Schaufeli, W. B. (2001). The job demands-resources model of burnout. *Journal of Applied Psychology, 86*(3), 499–512.

Diclemente, C. C., Marinilli, A. S., Singh, M., & Bellino, L. E. (2001). The role of feedback in the process of health behavior change. *American Journal of Health Behavior, 25*(3), 217–227.

Doumas, D. M., & Andersen, L. (2009). Reducing alcohol use in first-year university students: Evaluation of a web-based personalized feedback program. *Journal of College Counseling, 12*(1), 18–32.

European Framework Agreement on stress at work. (2004). Retrieved from http://www.worker-participation.eu/EU-Social-Dialogue/Interprofessional-ESD/Outcomes/Framework-agreements/Framework-agreement-on-stress-at-work-2004

Hackman, J. R., & Oldham, G. R. (1976). Motivation through the design of work: Test of a theory. *Organizational Behavior and Human Performance, 16*(2), 250–279.

Hackman, J. R., & Oldham, G. R. (1980). *Work redesign.* Reading, MA: Addison-Wesley.

Hakanen, J. J., Bakker, A. B., & Schaufeli, W. B. (2006). Burnout and work engagement among teachers. *Journal of School Psychology, 43*(6), 495–513.

Herzberg, F. I. (1966). *Work and the nature of man.* Cleveland, OH: Holland.

Karasek, R. A. (1979). Job demands, job decision latitude, and mental strain: Implications for job redesign. *Administrative Science Quarterly, 24*(2), 285–308.

Karasek, R. A., & Theorell, T. (1990). *Healthy work. Stress, productivity and the reconstruction of working life.* New York, NY: Basic Books.

Kurzman, P. A. (2013). Employee Assistance Programs for the new millennium: Emergence of the comprehensive model. *Social Work in Mental Health, 11*(5), 381–403.

Larimer, M. E., & Cronce, J. M. (2007). Identification, prevention and treatment revisited: Individual-focused college drinking prevention strategies 1999–2006. *Addictive Behaviors, 32,* 2439–2468.

Leslie, D. R., Holzhalb, C. M., & Holland, T. P. (1998). Measuring staff empowerment: Development of a worker empowerment scale. *Research on Social Work Practice, 8*(2), 212–222.

Maslach, C., & Leiter, M. P. (1997). *The truth about burnout: How organizations cause personal stress and what to do about it.* San Francisco, CA: Jossey Bass.

Maslach, C., Schaufeli, W. B., & Leiter, M. P. (2001). Job burnout. *Annual Review of Psychology, 52*(1), 397–422.

Roberts, K. H., & Glick, W. (1981). The job characteristics approach to task design: A critical review. *Journal of Applied Psychology, 66*(2), 193–217.

Roman, P. M., & Blum, T. C. (1985). The core technology of employee assistance programs. *The Almacan, 15*(3), 8–19.

Schaufeli, W. B., & Bakker, A. B. (2003). *Utrecht work engagement scale: Preliminary manual.* Utrecht, the Netherlands: Occupational Health Psychology Unit, Utrecht University.

Schmidt, U., Landau, S., Pombo-Carril, M. G., Bara-Carril, N., Reid, Y., Murray, K., . . . Katzman, M. (2006). Does personalized feedback improve the outcome of cognitive-behavioural guided self-care in bulimia nervosa? A preliminary randomized controlled trial. *British Journal of Clinical Psychology, 45*, 111–121.

Schmitz, G., & Schwarzer, R. (1999). Teachers' proactive attitude: Construct description and psychometric analyses. *Zeitschrift für Empirische Pädagogik, 13*(1), 3–27.

Schwarzer, R., & Jerusalem, M. (1995). Generalized self-efficacy scale. Measures in health psychology: A user's portfolio. *Causal and Control Beliefs, 1*, 35–37.

Siegrist, J. (1996). Adverse health effects of high-effort/low-reward conditions. *Journal of Occupational Health Psychology, 1*(1), 27–41.

Van Daele, T., Van Audenhove, C., Vansteenwegen, D., Hermans, D., & Van den Bergh, O. (2013). Effectiveness of a six session stress reduction program for groups. *Mental Health & Prevention, 1*(1), 19–25.

Vander Elst, T., Eertmans, A., Taeymans, S., De Witte, H., & De Cuyper, N. (2011). The Short Inventory on Stress and Well-being: A psychometric evaluation of the well-being indicators. *Romanian Journal of Applied Psychology, 13*(1), 1–10.

World Health Organization. (1946). *Preamble to the Constitution of the World Health Organization as adopted by the International Health Conference, New York, 19 June – 22 July 1946; signed on 22 July 1946 by the representatives of 61 States (Official Records of the World Health Organization, no. 2, p. 100) and entered into force on 7 April 1948.* Retrieved from http://www.who.int/about/definition/en/print.html

Evaluating EAP Counseling in the Chinese Workplace: A Study with a Brief Instrument

PEIZHONG LI, PhD

Chestnut Global Partners, China, Shanghai, China

DAVID A. SHARAR, PhD

Chestnut Global Partners, Bloomington, Illinois, USA

RICHARD LENNOX, PhD

Chestnut Global Partners, Hillsborough, North Carolina, USA

WEI ZHUANG, MS

University at Albany, State University of New York, Albany, New York, USA

This study examines if and to what degree an Employee Assistance Program (EAP) intervention improves Chinese employees' workplace functioning. The sample included 670 employees from 26 local and multinational companies in China who received EAP counseling. The Chinese translation of the Workplace Outcome Suite-Short Version, a five-item outcome assessment instrument, was used as a pre/post measure. Four of the five items showed significant improvements from the pre- to posttest. The effect sizes on the items varied, indicating that EAP produced different levels of impact on dimensions of workplace functioning. Future research should examine the influences of different EAP models, client organizations, and dimensions of workplace functioning.

INTRODUCTION

Employee Assistance Program (EAP) has become widely accepted among employers in the United States. Most large and midsize employers in the United States provide EAP services as a prepaid benefit to help employees and their families with a variety of personal concerns that may have negative effects on job performance (Masi, 2004). In emerging markets such as China, EAP has been introduced recently as a result of rapid economic development and integration with the global economy. International EAPs have set up operations in China either independently or in joint ventures with local partners (Shi, 2006). Meanwhile, "home-grown" EAPs of various sizes and levels of expertise have sprang up in China's major economic centers (Wang, 2005; Zhang, 2006). On the client side, large multinational and state-owned companies lead the way to purchase EAP services for their employees (Shi, 2006).

At the conceptual core of EAP counseling is a focus on the impact of the employee's unresolved personal problems on work effectiveness and occupational functioning (Roman, 1981). This focus on workplace outcomes differentiates EAP counseling from the traditional "psychotherapeutic" perspective; it calls for measures of service effectiveness. Moreover, these measures must capture whether EAPs achieve results relevant to workplace effectiveness, and thus meaningful to employer representatives or stake-holders in Human Resources, Employee Benefits, and Occupational Health and Safety. This focus on job-related outcomes requires EAP providers to scrutinize the end results of their intervention, especially the effects that employers care about, for example, less absenteeism and presenteeism, higher levels of work engagement, and lower levels of distress at work. The need for accurate, targeted, and timely assessment of EAP effectiveness is particularly strong in emerging markets such as China, where the concepts and practices of EAP are beginning to be accepted by employers and employees but have not taken roots as in North America and Europe (Wang, 2005; Zhang, 2006).

THE STATUS OF EAP OUTCOME RESEARCH

In 1988, Pallassana Balgopal, a veteran occupational social worker and researcher, pointed out that the "growth of EAPs has not been accompanied by an increase in rigorous evaluation of these programs" (Balgopal & Patchner, 1988, p. 17). This statement remains accurate over two decades later. Even in more mature markets such as the United States, assessment of EAP effectiveness has ample room for progress. Typical measures of an EAP focus on process metrics such as utilization rates, presenting problems, and demographics. These measures fail to demonstrate the program's actual effectiveness in obtaining a positive outcome in the workplace. Ironically, most EAP providers do not quantify their impact on the field's original claim—that when employees' personal and employers' job performance concerns overlap, EAPs improve job performance. The following commonly used measures of effectiveness fall short of this goal.

1. Measures of client satisfaction. Many EAP counselors are likable and caring, therefore may be rated positively by clients that have experienced little or no change in their work environment.
2. Case studies or testimonials. Employees' first-hand, positive anecdotal accounts of personal experiences with EAP are valuable but imprecise; they are not standardized, quantifiable, or reliable outcome indicators. They have limited impact when used to demonstrate the business-relevant value of EAP to Finance, Benefits, Human Resources, or Medical personnel.
3. Utilization rates. A "high" utilization rate is often interpreted as indicating that the EAP must be successful. However, in reality it indicates the extent to which employees use the EAP, not if the EAP has had a positive workplace impact.

Much of the evidence on EAP's efficacy for improving workplace functioning sits in non-peer-reviewed outlets, such as proprietary internal evaluations, conference presentations, and trade magazine articles (Attridge, 2010). The methodological quality of the research and credibility of claims in these outlets are either weak or unknown (Arthur, 2001; Attridge, 2010; Pompe & Sharar, 2008).

Only a small number of EAP outcome studies have been published in peer-reviewed journals. Attridge (2010) pointed out that the small scientific literature showing positive organizational impact of EAP is unrepresentative of the situation of the industry in the types of cases presented by the clients as well as the interventions offered by EAPs. These studies tend to focus on minor subsets of EAP cases with serious mental health or alcohol abuse issues. The type of EAP intervention used with these serious cases involved the usual assessment and brief counseling components but with the critical addition of long-term follow-up, active case management, and frequent collaboration with treatment providers and referral sources. However, most contemporary EAPs serve a diverse clientele. The majority of typical cases is less clinically severe and only receives brief counseling within the EAP, that is, six sessions or less with no onward referral for longer-term treatment outside the EAP and into the medical plan benefit (Sharar, 2009). It is unclear if the prevalent "brief counseling only" type of cases in EAP would yield the same outcomes or cost-offsets as the older "core technology" style programs that focused on intensive case management and follow-up with more severe, high-risk cases.

Another limit to the current research in EAP effectiveness is the cultural-specific nature of the studies. Most of the studies have been done in North America, where EAP has had a relatively long history. The typical research participants are employees from organizations in the United States or Canada. The same findings may not be replicated in countries with different cultures, customs and levels of economic development. As EAP providers expand their businesses into emerging markets such as China, there is a strong need to understand how well their model works in an environment where the concepts and practices of EAP or any form of mental health care are relatively new, the training and licensing systems for mental health professionals are relatively weak, and the prevalent attitudes toward psychological issues and their management or resolution differ from Western societies (Lim, Lim, Michael, Cai, & Schock, 2010).

SEARCH FOR A NIMBLE INSTRUMENT

The reasons that the EAP field has not produced adequate outcomes research are many. These include (1) the lack of a short, valid, relevant, and affordable measure; (2) little or no cooperation from employers; (3) no extra funding or fee increases to implement credible evaluations; (4) problems in getting staff to reliably collect data; (5) lack of in-house scientific expertise to analyze data; (6) the highly competitive and proprietary nature of EAP that does not emphasize or reward the integration of research & practice (Sharar, Pompe, & Lennox, 2013). To overcome some of the above difficulties in measuring the effects of EAP intervention, researchers need a short instrument and nimble data collection methods that minimize the intrusiveness for help-seeking employees and client organizations but still yield reliable results in an economic manner.

The Workplace Outcome Suite (WOS) is an instrument specifically designed for quick and reliable assessment of EAP effectiveness (Lennox, Sharar, Schmitz, & Goehner, 2010). It measures those outcomes that are likely to show change if the intervention works. It is short, psychometrically tested and validated, workplace focused, and easy to administer (Lennox et al., 2010). Two validation studies have tested the reliability of the scales, structural validity of the items, and construct validity of the unit-weighted scale scores. These studies support the use of WOS to evaluate the workplace effects of EAP counseling (Lennox et al., 2010). The original WOS contains five scales that measure constructs central to understanding EAP effectiveness: Absenteeism, Presenteeism, Work Engagement, Life Satisfaction, and Workplace Distress. Each scale includes five items, thus a total of 25 items in the suite. Lennox et al. (2010) recently developed a shorter version of WOS (WOS-Short), with only one item on each of the five scales, thus five items in total. This brief instrument opens new possibilities for researchers and EAP providers to evaluate the effects of EAP counseling on the various aspects of employee functioning in a cost-efficient and reliable manner.

THE CURRENT STUDY

The objective of this outcome study is to examine if and to what degree EAP counseling improves workplace functioning in China. Employees' workplace effectiveness was measured with the Chinese translation of the WOS-Short before and after counseling to examine whether they improved on the job. The single-group pre-test–post-test design is common when a matched comparison group is not available or permitted. In this study it was selected because it would avoid disrupting the participants' normal help-seeking process, thus minimizing the burden on the employees and client organization. The research hypothesis was that the participants would show better workplace functioning after EAP counseling compared with before the intervention. With this design, the investigators' intent was not to authoritatively explain why employees have improved at work, or prove that EAP services have caused the improvements. However, showing that EAP service is consistently associated with improved work effectiveness supports the hypothesis that EAP contributes to improved work effectiveness.

METHOD

Research Participants

The participants were 670 full-time employees from 26 local and multinational companies located in different regions in China. These companies use the same external EAP vendor in China. The sample included only employees, whereas family members were excluded. The participants received EAP counseling between May 2012 and July 2013.

Assessment Instrument

The WOS-Short has five items measuring different dimensions of workplace functioning. The item on absenteeism is an open-ended question asking the employee to report the total number of hours missed due to personal problems within the last month. The remaining four items use 5-point Likert-type rating scales for employees to evaluate their functioning within the last month. The item on presenteeism asks the employee to rate the degree to which personal problems keep the employee from concentrating on work. It measures productivity decrements while the employee is present but not working at his or her optimum due to unresolved personal problems. The item on work engagement asks the employee to rate the degree to which the employee is "often eager to get to the work site to start the day." It measures the extent to which the employee is invested in or passionate about the job. Workplace problems are likely to diminish when employees are highly engaged or enthusiastic about their work. The item on life satisfaction asks the employee to rate the degree to which "life seems to be going very well." This is a global measure of the impact of work and life issues on one's sense of well-being. Finally, the Workplace Distress scale asks the employee to rate the degree to which the employee dreads going to work. Employees seek EAP service because they are distressed about something, which makes them less effective at work.

The WOS-Short was translated from its English original into simplified Chinese. One of the authors, a Chinese-English bilingual with a master's degree in psychology from a U.S. university first translated the instrument. Another author, a Chinese-English bilingual with a doctoral degree in psychology from a U.S. university reviewed the translation and suggested amendments. Disagreements between them were resolved through discussions. Then five psychologists with masters' degrees evaluated the Chinese translation for clarity, understandability, and face validity. Disagreements generated in this process were resolved through discussions. The instrument was subsequently pilot-tested with Chinese staff and employees before being put into production. The finalized Chinese Translation of WOS-Short (WOS-Short, Chinese) was used in this study for measuring workplace functioning before and after EAP counseling.

The Intervention – EAP Counseling

Sharar (2009) found that counselors use a variety of assessment and therapeutic approaches with EAP cases. Some of these approaches are more empirically supported than others. In the Chinese context, the lack of control and standardization in the methods of EAP counseling is even more prominent. The concepts and practices of mental health counseling have a relatively short history, with a professional licensing system introduced only in 2002 (Lim et al., 2010). The training, regulation, and supervision system in the country is still evolving (Lim et al., 2010). Counselors licensed for providing psychological interventions come from a variety of educational and professional backgrounds. This situation limits the pool of qualified staff and affiliate counselors available to primary EAP vendors in China. Moreover, local and international EAPs of various sizes have different operation processes and standards.

The EAP provider in this study is a joint-venture between a U.S. EAP and Chinese partners. Its services are modeled after the U.S. EAP, which provides training and supervising. The counselors in this study included staff and affiliates. Their approaches may be best described as brief or short-term counseling. This means that there is an emphasis on being helpful in six or fewer sessions, identifying specific problem areas and using direct intervention techniques. Given the varied approaches and competencies among the counselors, the "EAP counseling" intervention deployed in this study is not strictly defined or specified. The lack of control over the method of interventions is out of necessity and by design; it provides an opportunity to assess EAP outcomes in a natural and realistic setting in China.

Procedure

Employees seeking EAP services received assessment with the WOS-Short, Chinese twice, that is, before introducing counseling and about 90 days after completing counseling. Ninety-day follow-up was set as a procedure to allow EAP counseling to run its usual course and have potential for sustained impact. The pre-test was conducted as part of the routine telephonic intake, before counseling was set up with a staff or affiliate. Recruitment involved asking clients who called EAP to voluntarily participate in the evaluation, followed by verbal informed consent and guarantees of confidentiality. Less than 5% of clients declined to participate or dropped out after pre-test. During the pre-test, intake counselors let clients know that a staff person would follow-up with them in about 90 days to complete the post-test. Complete locator information was gathered (e-mail, cell, work, home phone) to help increase response rates. The post-test was administered over the phone. Follow-up staff made up to three attempts to reach each client and gather data before eliminating the client from the sample. No more than three follow-up attempts occurred to minimize potential complaints about the process. In all cases, the completed pre- and post-tests were linked with a common identification number and each client's data were placed and stored on a single line organized in an Excel spreadsheet. These Excel files were then transferred into a statistical package (SPSS version 19) for statistical analysis.

RESULTS

In the combined sample, 32.09% of participants were male, 62.42% were female and 1.49% did not report gender. This gender makeup reflects the typical situation of EAP use in China. The male and female participants did not differ on the pre- and post-test scores except for the post-test work engagement. Therefore gender was not included in further analyses on the dimensions of intervention outcomes except for work engagement.

We examined whether the employees improved on the five items of the WOS-Short, Chinese from before to after counseling and compared the results with a study in the United States with the five-item, five-scale full version of WOS (Sharar et al., 2013) where applicable. We also examined the effect sizes of the pre-test/post-test comparisons to understand to what degrees EAP improved workplace functioning.

Improvement on Absenteeism

The distributions of the absenteeism scores were highly skewed. The majority of the respondents had extremely low scores, whereas a small minority had high scores on pre- and post-tests. More specifically, 70.60% and 86.42% of the participants reported missing no work in the pre- and post-test, respectively, whereas the maximum hours of missed work for the pre- and post-test were both 100. The means for the pre- and post-tests were less than their associated standard deviations (Table 1), indicating that the left-censored distribution had most of its observation near the lower end of the scale. Similar skewed distributions on absenteeism scores were found in the U.S. study with the full version of WOS (Sharar et al., 2013).

Because the skewed distributions violated the normality assumption underlying parametric tests, a Wilcoxon signed-rank test was used for hypothesis testing. The hours of missed work decreased from pre- to post-test (Table 1). This difference was statistically significant, $Z = 8.49$, $p < .001$ (two-tailed); the employees missed fewer hours of work after EAP counseling.

Improvements on the Likert-Type Scales

Pre- and post-test scores on the Likert-type scales for the remaining items of WOS-Short, Chinese showed approximately normal distributions and posed little risk for t tests. The mean scores on presenteeism decreased substantially from pre- to post-test (Table 1). A paired-sample t test showed that the difference was statistically significant, $t(669) = 19.71$, $p < 0.001$ (all t tests are two-tailed); Presenteeism improved after EAP counseling. The scores on Life Satisfaction increased substantially from pre- to post-test (Table 1). A paired-sample t test showed that this difference was statistically significant, $t(669) = -14.54$, $p < 0.001$; the employees' evaluation of their quality of life

TABLE 1 Chinese Employees' Scores on Workplace Outcome Suite-Short, Chinese Before and After Employee Assistance Program Counseling

	Pre-test		Post-test		
Item	M	SD	M	SD	N
Absenteeism	2.63	8.97	0.79	4.83	670
Presenteeism	3.14	1.38	2.02	1.18	670
Work engagement	3.06	1.35	3.09	1.34	670
Life satisfaction	3.01	1.29	3.72	1.08	670
Workplace distress	1.78	1.17	1.49	0.94	670

improved after EAP counseling. The scores on workplace distress decreased from pre- to post-test (Table 1). A paired-sample t test showed that this difference was statistically significant $t(669) = 6.39, p < 0.001$; the employees felt less distressed at work after EAP counseling. Because men and women differed on work engagement in the post-test, we included gender in the analysis of change from pre- to post-test on this item. We performed a two-by-two mixed factorial analysis of variance (ANOVA) with gender (male and female) as a between-group variable and work engagement scores for the pre- and post-test as repeated measures. The repeated measures at pre- and post-test had no main effect, $F(1, 658) = 1.22, p > 0.05$, indicating that as a whole the employees (men and women combined) had no significant change from pre- to post-test on work engagement (see Table 1 for the means). The interaction between the repeated measures of pre- and post-test and gender was not significant either, $F(1, 658) = 2.51, p > 0.05$, indicating that men and women had the same pattern of results from pre- to post-test, that is, no improvement. It is worth noting that this pattern of results was also found in the U.S. study with the full version of WOS (Sharar et al., 2013); the U.S. participants also showed no change on work engagement but significant improvement on the other WOS subscales. The only significant effect in the ANOVA was the main effect for gender, $F(1, 658) = 6.82, p < 0.05$. The men had higher work engagement scores than women in the pre- ($Ms = 3.16$ and 3.00) and post-tests ($Ms = 3.32$ and 2.98). The gender difference at the pre-test did not reach conventional level of statistical significance, $t(658) = 1.32$, $p > 0.05$, whereas the gender difference at post-test was statistically significant, $t(658) = 3.09, p < 0.05$.

Effect Size Analyses

Researchers and client organizations are interested in not only whether an EAP intervention has any effect, but also how big the effect is, whether it is small, medium, or large. The size of the effect is related to the return on investments. This information is not available from the statistics for hypothesis testing (Thompson, 2006; Volker, 2006). A small p value means that the difference between the pre- and post-tests has a low likelihood for being due to random error. However, it does not tell us how big the difference is. A small difference could show up as statistically significant in the p value for a variety of reasons. Conversely, a large effect could fail to reach the 0.05 cutoff point (Durlak, 2009). For example in this study, the various types and severity of problems clients bring to EAP and the diverse methods of counseling could introduce measurement errors and increase the likelihood that that we would fail to reject the null hypothesis and make Type II errors. On the other hand, the effect size provides an estimate of how large the effect is.

We computed the effect sizes for the pre- and post-test differences on the WOS-Short, Chinese items using the method described by Lipsey and

Wilson (2001), that is, dividing the difference between the pre- and post-test means by the pre-test standard deviation (see also Durlak, 2009). We used Cohen (1988)'s classic rule of the thumb (0.20, 0.50, and 0.80 for small, medium, and large effects, respectively) for interpreting the results, because there is no literature on the typical effect size for EAP intervention. The results indicate that EAP intervention produced effects of various sizes on the five items of the instrument. Large and medium effect sizes were observed for presenteeism ($d = 0.81$) and life satisfaction ($d = 0.55$), whereas small effect sizes were observed for workplace distress ($d = 0.25$) and absenteeism ($d = 0.21$). No effect was observed on work engagement. These results indicate that EAP counseling had different levels of influence on aspects of workplace functioning. Moreover, as an assessment instrument WOS-Short, Chinese has not only picked up the subtle effects of intervention, but also differentiated effects of various sizes.

DISCUSSION

The EAP field faces a global need for empirical assessment of the impact of its services. In the United States, with an increased focus on "comparative effectiveness" research to identify which health and welfare benefits work best for which patients under what circumstances, the EAP field can no longer avoid scrutiny of its methods for gauging effectiveness (Sharar et al., 2013). In emerging markets such as China, where employers and employees alike have just begun to be exposed to EAP services, more precise, targeted, and timely assessments of the effectiveness of EAP services are equally important (Wang, 2005; Zhang, 2006).

Taken together, the results of this study support the hypothesis that EAP counseling produces positive changes to Chinese employees' workplace adjustment. Significant changes have occurred in the hypothesized direction on four of the five items of the WOS-Short, Chinese. Moreover, these changes persisted 90 days after the employees received brief counseling, indicating that the effects of EAP intervention were lasting and sustainable. The finding that not all items of the WOS-Short, Chinese showed identical changes is unsurprising given the multi-dimensional nature of the workplace outcomes measured in the instrument. This pattern of results shows that the instrument addresses similar yet distinct constructs and has some levels of discriminant validity.

Effect size analyses provide more nuanced information on the efficacy of EAP counseling in the various aspects of workplace adjustment. For the Chinese employees, EAP produced larger effects in reducing presenteeism and improving life satisfaction than lowering absenteeism and workplace distress and promoting work engagement. These levels of improvement should be viewed in the context that EAP counseling is brief and rarely provides protocol-driven interventions. Instead, counselors rely on their own clinical insights and highly varied approaches to intervene with clients' presenting problems (Sharar, 2009; Sharar et al., 2013). This situation is particularly serious in an emerging market like China, where training, licensing, and supervision of counselors are less developed and uneven (Lim et al., 2010). Despite the complexities and drawbacks, EAP counseling produced lasting improvements for Chinese employees, an encouraging sign for EAPs and client organizations.

A cautionary note on the interpretation of effect size is in order. The effect size of a particular study is affected by the design characteristics. A questionnaire study is likely to underestimate the effect size compared with controlled experiments. Without existing literature on the typical effect sizes for EAP intervention, the effect sizes in this study should be considered as relative rather than absolute. Moreover, effect size should not be confused with the importance of the intervention; it must be viewed within the context of the practical implications on employees' workplace functioning. This point is particularly important to bear in mind when doing applied research in natural settings.

Work engagement turned out to be an area that seemed resistant to change for the Chinese workers in this study and U.S. employees in Sharar et al. (2013). Different interpretations for this result are plausible. Maybe employees' workplace engagement is particularly difficult to change. Maybe EAP counselors are inadequately equipped to help clients love their jobs more and are not in a position to directly change any environmental conditions in the work environment. Further studies are needed to examine what types of EAP interventions are effective for what types of workplace adjustment issues. An interesting finding with respect to Chinese employees' work engagement is that men scored higher, a gender difference that is independent from the EAP intervention. This result is compatible with the Chinese society's traditional gender roles; work is more important for men than women in creating a sense of personal success, value, and self-worth. The fact that WOS-short, Chinese has picked up this subtle difference offers support for its sensitivity.

The results of this study have important implications for measuring correlated but distinct workplace outcomes with a short instrument. Conventional wisdom believes that short scales lack reliability and thus provide underpowered tests of intervention effectiveness. In this study the WOS-Short, Chinese successfully identified significant changes in most of the variables under statistically underpowered conditions. It is worth noting that Sharar et al. (2013) obtained the same pattern of results with U.S. employees using the full version of WOS. There is reason to believe that WOS-Short can serve as an effective and reliable tool for assessing EAP outcomes.

This is the first published study to measure the workplace effects of EAP intervention in China. The study should be replicated among other EAPs and include employers of different types, such as foreign-owned and multi-national companies operating in China. Moreover, this kind of outcome evaluation should be a routine form of monitoring among China employers who purchase EAPs.

REFERENCES

Attridge, M. (2010). Taking the pareto path to ROI. *Journal of Employee Assistance, 40*(3), 12–15.

Arthur, A. (2001, July-August). Employee assistance programs: Do they work? *EAP Association Exchange, 31*(4), 21–23.

Balgopal, P., & Patchner, M. (1988). Evaluating employee assistance programs: Obstacles, issues, and strategies. *Employee Assistance Quarterly, 3*(3–4), 95–105.

Cohen, J. (1988). *Statistical power analysis for the behavioral sciences* (2nd ed.). Hilllsdale, NJ: Erlbaum.

Durlak, J. A. (2009). How to select, calculate, and interpret effect sizes. *Journal of Pediatric Psychology, 34*(9), 917–928.

Lennox, R., Sharar, D., Schmitz, E., & Goehner, D. (2010). Development and validation of the Chestnut Global Partners Workplace Outcome Suite. *Journal of Workplace Behavioral Health, 25*(2), 107–131.

Lim, S., Lim, B. K. H., Michael, R., Cai, R., & Schock, C. K. (2010). The trajectory of counseling in China: Past, present, and future trends. *Journal of Counseling & Development, 88*, 4–8.

Lipsey, M. W., & Wilson, D. B. (2001). *Practical meta-analysis.* Thousand Oaks, CA: Sage.

Masi, D. (2004). EAPs in the year 2002. In R. Manderscheid & M. Henderson (Eds.), *Mental health, United States* (DHHS Pub No. SMA 3938, pp. 209–223). Rockville, MD: Substance Abuse Mental Health Services Administration.

Pompe, J., & Sharar, D. (2008). Preparing for the challenges of research. *Journal of Employee Assistance, 38*(2), 7–9.

Roman, P. (1981). From employee alcoholism to employee assistance. *Journal of Studies on Alcohol, 42*(3), 244–272.

Sharar, D. (2009). General mental health practitioners as EAP network affiliates: Does short-term counseling overlap with general practice psychotherapy? *Brief Treatment and Crisis Intervention, 8*(4), 358–369.

Sharar, D. A., Pompe, J., & Lennox, R. (2013). *Evaluating the workplace effects of EAP counseling.* Unpublished manuscript. Chestnut Global Partners, Bloomington, Illinois.

Shi, K. (2006). Yuan Gong Yuan Zhu Ji Hua Zai Zhong Guo De Fa Zhan Yu Si Kao [Observations on the development of employee assistance program in China]. *Xinziben, 3*, 14–17.

Thompson, B. (2006). Research synthesis: Effect sizes. In J. L. Green, G. Camilli, & P. B. Elmore (Eds.), *Handbook of complementary methods in educational research* (pp. 583–603). Mahwah, NJ: Erlbaum.

Volker, M. A. (2006). Reporting effect sizes in school psychology research. *Psychology in the Schools, 43*, 653–672.

Wang, Y. (2005). Yuan Gong Bang Zhu Ji Hua Zai Wo Guo De Fa Zhan He Qian Jing [The current status of future prospects of EAP in China]. *Rencaikaifa, 6,* 10–11.

Zhang, X. (2006). Yuan Gong Bang Zhu Ji Hua, Zhong Guo EAP De Li Lun Yu Shi Jian [Employee assistance programs: Theories and practice of Chinese EAP]. Beijing, China: Publishing House of Chinese Academy of Social Sciences.

Eureka: An Employee Services Perception Study in Continental Europe

DEBORA VANSTEENWEGEN, PhD

ISW Limits, Leuven, Belgium

MANUEL SOMMER, PhD

Clinica CAPA and Psychology Department, CIP-UAL, Lisbon, Portugal

DIRK ANTONISSEN, MA

ISW Limits, Leuven, Belgium

TITO LANEIRO, PhD, and ODETE NUNES, PhD

Psychology Department, CIP-UAL, Lisbon, Portugal

The EUREKA research study, based on an originally developed comprehensive Employee Services Questionnaire, assessed current and desired services in the Employee Assistance (EA) field in six Eurozone countries (three northern European countries [Belgium, France, and The Netherlands] and three southern European countries [Portugal, Spain, and Greece]). A total of 327 participants completed the online questionnaire. Several relevant and interesting findings about the prevalence and needs of EA-type services in several industry grouping and different cultural settings could be determined. These results can help shape the responses from Employee Assistance Program providers attending to different European cultural and economic realities.

Color versions of one or more of the figures in the article can be found online at www.tandfonline.com/wjwb.

INTRODUCTION

Through the approval of the European Pact for Mental Health and Well-Being at the European Union high-level conference in Brussels (June, 2008), the European Commission stressed the importance of mental health and well-being for its member states, stakeholders and citizens. The 2000 report of the International Labour Organization (ILO) and the World Health Organization (WHO) in Geneva on "Mental health and work: Impact, issues and good practices" (Harnois & Gabriel, 2000) reviews many good mental health work-place practices and explicitly mentions the importance of Employee Assistance Programs (EAPs).

Although there is a clear interest in mental health services at the workplace, it is clear that the Employee Assistance (EA) business in Europe is not well-developed yet and lacks a good model of EAP that is specifically tailored to the needs of European employees and employers. The landscape on mental health and well-being at the workplace is very diverse (Bhagat, Steverson, & Segovis, 2007). Different countries have different intervention cultures and different professionals have been involved in working with mental health and well-being in the workplace. Therefore a good view on the needs with regard to employee services in continental Europe is wel-come. The European needs might be rather different than the dominant needs in the United States. To survive, not to become a commodity and to flourish in Europe, EAP providers will need to show some flexibility and creativity in how they present and develop their mental health services toward companies. Also special attention should be given to the large cul-tural diversity present in continental Europe implying that the context and the actual embedding of EA services in the different countries in Europe might differ largely and tailored solutions might be necessary.

In this study, it was investigated to what extent and under which form EA services are currently available in companies in continental Europe and what the needs of employers/Human Resource (HR) managers and employ-ees are with regard to these services. Because our focus is on potential future directions and new developments in the field of EAP, we explicitly wanted to take an open and nonbiased perspective on EA services. Because the large cultural diversity and the fact that EAP provided by an external organization is not a common practice in most European countries, we avoided setting up our research relying on a narrow definition of what EAP is and which ser-vices it should include. In contrast, we started with a very broad range of employee services that could be delivered by an external partner including typical EAP-services viewed from a U.S./U.K. perspective but also some other mental-health related services such as training, online assessment, HR advice, and so on.

When starting with a wide list of services, an important additional issue to take into account is whether these services are or should be delivered by an external organization and thus are relevant for the EA business or not. In many companies in Europe mental health issues are taken up by internal structures or persons such as a medical doctor, person of trust, psychologist, or social worker. When investigating the market opportunities for the different services, it is therefore of crucial importance that we get information about whether these services are currently externally provided and whether respondents think an external partner to deliver the service would be preferable.

Systematic research that reviews the EAP field in Europe is very limited. One of the few studies available is the Buon and Taylor study (2007). In this study 103 HR managers coming from the United Kingdom, Denmark, and Germany (& Switzerland) were asked about the value of EAPs. In this study, we wanted to more systematically cover the diversity present in Continental Europe, and we decided to set up our research in three northern and three southern countries that were not earlier included in the Buon and Taylor study. We selected Belgium, The Netherlands, and France as the three northern countries and Spain, Portugal, and Greece as the three southern countries.

Furthermore, in each of these countries we wanted to reach employers/HR managers as well as employees. Both might have a different perspective on employee services with regard to satisfaction with the services as well as with the perceived needs. Most research so far directs its attention toward the HR managers who are usually the buyers of EAPs and take up the responsibility within the company for the well-being policy. However the employees might reveal additional information as they are the end users of the employee services and might be more sensitive with regard to the specific needs at the work floor.

With regard to the size of the companies, we aimed at a representative sample for those companies usually having structural EA services available. The larger the companies the more the chance that they have these services provided by an external partner. Therefore a larger representation of medium-sized to large companies is preferable in this sample. With regard to the industry grouping we hope to end up with a sample that is representative for the different sectors. If not, a weighing of the sample data can be considered. The statistics made available through Eurostat will be used as a reference to compare our sample.[1]

METHOD

In line with the exploratory nature of our research and to guarantee cost and time efficiency, we decided to use a survey research methodology. After a small pilot study ($N = 50$ coming mainly from Belgium and Portugal) to check the reliability of the questionnaire, an online link toward the online questionnaire was send out to employees and HR managers in three northern

(Belgium, The Netherlands, and France) and three southern (Greece, Portugal, and Spain) countries in Europe. We used a snowball sampling method with quota for the number of HR managers and employees in each country. Personal as well as business contacts of the broad network of the investigators as well as the network of the Employee Assistance European Forum (EAEF) and some EA partners and providers in the European Union (EU) were used to send the questionnaire around. Because of expected difficulties in translation and back-translation and additional problems of generalizability over the six countries, it was decided to develop the questionnaire in English only. Familiarity with the English language was thus a prerequisite to be included in this study.

Furthermore, the Employee Services Questionnaire[2] was developed. The first part contained some basic questions about the company and the respondents' position in the company. The respondent had to indicate gender, country (Belgium, The Netherlands, Spain, Portugal, France, or Greece), the size of the company in number of employees, industry grouping (open question), staff category (blue collar, white collar, executives, management/board, other), working in the HR department (yes or no), the number of people directly under supervision, and whether their company had a duty-to-care policy.

For the remainder of the questionnaire, a list of employee services was created. Starting from the list of services that were included in the Buon and Taylor (2007) study, we divided our list in two parts. The first part focused on the content of the services such as trauma, alcohol and drugs, depression and anxiety, and the second part contained questions about not only how the services are delivered (face-to-face, telephone, and e-mail online) but also whether services should be available for family members. This resulted in a list of 18 different services content wise. All the Buon and Taylor services were included but two services were moved to the second part mainly containing a method (telephone counseling and services for family members) and two specific services were added: counseling for stress and motivational problems and counseling for depression, anxiety, and panic.

This list of 18 services was followed by eight questions about how these services are made available: through a website, brochures, personal contact with a counselor by phone, e-mail or chat, training about assertiveness and communication, work–life, stress and healthy lifestyle, a 24/7 hotline, online assessment, and treatment programs and services for family members.

For HR managers, the list was extended by four questions about advice by consultants/external companies about how to set up mental health and well-being services within their company about communication/ sensibilization, about organizational surveys/audits, stress/health/well-being policy, and action plans to improve well-being.

These 30 services for HR managers and 26 for non-HR managers were presented twice sequentially in the same questionnaire to our respondents.

During the first presentation, we addressed the current situation: they had to indicate whether each service was currently present within their company (yes or no), whether the service was delivered by an internal or an external provider, and to what extent they were satisfied with these services on a 7-point Likert-type scale anchored 1 (*not at all*) to 7 (*very much*).

We explicitly mentioned what we meant by externally or internally delivered services. An *external person/partner* refers to an external consultant/EAP provider or psychologist/psychiatrist. An internal person or partner is an internal HR person, psychologist, social worker, medical doctor, or person of trust.

During the second presentation, we addressed the needs and asked to what extent do you think this service is important/useful on a 7-point Likert-type scale from 1 (*not at all useful*) to 7 (*very much*) and whether they would prefer an external/internal person/partner to deliver the service.

Sample Description

In total 327 participants (156 male and 171 female) completed our online questionnaire. Our sample represents three northern and three southern countries. In Figure 1 the distribution over the different countries is presented. In general, 198 employees (61%) were reached and 129 HR managers (39%).

In our sample, one half of the respondents are employees (with an over-representation of white-collar workers) and the other half are persons with responsibility within the company as 44% of our sample indicates to be part of the management/board of the company or an executive (see Fig. 2).

A similar pattern shows the number of persons that our respondents have under direct supervision (see Figure 3). In our sample the group of

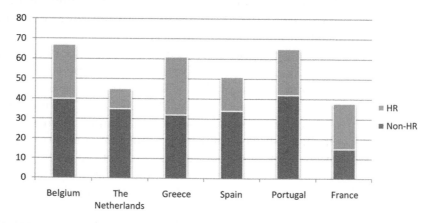

FIGURE 1 Number of respondents for each country divided in employees (non-Human Resource [HR]) and HR-managers.

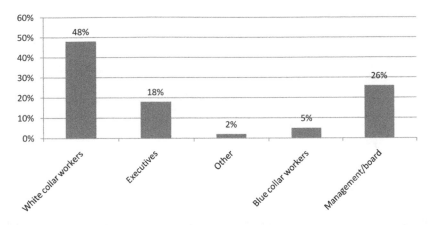

FIGURE 2 Distribution of the sample in percentages over the five staff categories.

respondents that have more than six persons under supervision is largely represented compared with the benchmark of ISW Limits (spin-off of Leuven University).[3] Again, this indicates that our sample contains a large share of persons with responsibility within the companies.

In Europe,[4] 92% of all enterprises have less than 10 employees (micro), 7% are small companies, and 1% are of medium size (between 50 and 249 employees). Only 0.2% of all companies have more than 250 employees. The latter group of large companies is responsible for a share of 33% of the active workforce. Medium companies employ 20% of the workforce and the small and microcompanies are together respectively responsible for 21% and 29% of the workforce. This distribution is not really different for the six countries included in this study except for the fact that the share of the microcompanies is a bit larger in the southern countries (Spain, Portugal, and Greece).

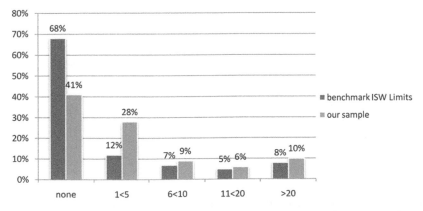

FIGURE 3 Distribution of this sample ($N = 327$) and the benchmark of ISW Limits (spin-off of Leuven University) with regard to the number of employees under direct supervision.

71

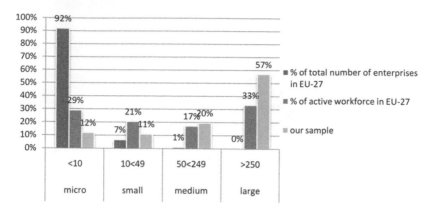

FIGURE 4 Percentage micro, small, medium, and large size companies of the total number of enterprises in the European Union-27 member countries (EU-27; dark blue bars) of the active workforce in the EU-27 (lighter blue bars) and the distribution in this sample (very light blue bars).

When comparing with the distribution of the active workforce that is employed by the different type of companies, it is clear that our sample contains an over-representation of large companies (57%) and an under-representation of microcompanies (see Fig. 4). However from the perspective of EAP, micro or small companies will barely have resources (interest, budget, etc.) for setting up structural EAP services, meaning that our sample represents the EA market as described in previous research in Europe (see Reddy, 2005; Hopkins, 2005) rather well.

Looking at the industry grouping represented in our sample, Figure 5 compares our sample with the distribution of the different sectors in the EU. The data sample of this study can be considered as representative for the

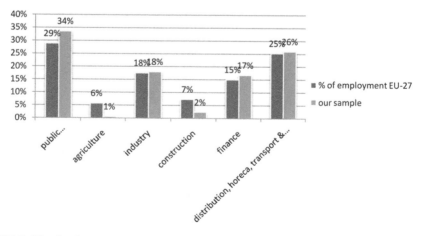

FIGURE 5 Distribution in percentages over the six large industry groupings for the sample compared to the percentage of the total employment in the European Union 27 member countries.

general situation in the EU. Although the numbers below represent the total group of European countries, it can be useful to keep in mind that for some countries the distribution might slightly deviate from the general European picture.[5] For France in particular the financial sector is larger than the EU mean. In Greece distribution takes a larger share, in Spain construction, and in Portugal and France category 1 (administration, health, & services) contains significantly more than the indicated 25% of the employment.

RESULTS

Current Status: List of Services

For each service, it is indicated in Table 1 to what extent these services are currently present within the companies of our respondents. The percentage of "yes" responses is given together with the valid N and the corresponding standard deviation. In Table 2, answers to the question "Is the current service provided internally of externally" are summarized. The proportion of companies that have the service provided by an external person or organization is indicated. Note that only the participants that indicated "yes" to the previous question were asked to fill in this question. This explains the low number of respondents for these specific questions in the table. In Table 3, the mean satisfaction score is presented for each service. Respondents had to indicate to what extent they were satisfied with the current services on a 7-point Likert-type scale from 1 (*not at all*) to 7 (*very much*).

TABLE 1 Valid N, Percentage Currently Present, and Standard Deviation for the List of 18 Employee Services

Current status presence	Valid N	% present	SD
Counseling_depressive, panic, or anxiety	304	50.7	50.1
Counseling_stress & motivation	296	49.7	50.1
Alcohol & other drug	283	31.8	46.7
Critical incident and trauma	285	36.8	48.3
Internet based (online) counseling	281	14.2	35.0
Financial/legal	278	51.1	50.1
Work–life	277	35.7	48.0
Childcare/eldercare services	275	18.2	38.6
Expatriate support services	275	34.9	47.8
Concierge services	274	23.7	42.6
Coaching	276	61.2	48.8
Human Resource consultation	276	75.7	43.0
Performance management	276	64.5	47.9
Management training	275	66.5	47.3
Other specialist training (healthy lifestyle)	276	27.9	44.9
Stress management	275	25.5	43.6
Harassment, bullying, or grievance investigation	276	40.9	49.3
Workplace mediation	274	29.9	45.9

TABLE 2 Valid N, Percentage Provided Externally, and Standard Deviation for the List of 18 Employee Services

Current status external	Valid N	% external	SD
Counseling_depressive, panic, or anxiety	154	53.2	50.1
Counseling_stress & motivation	143	46.2	50.0
Alcohol & other drug	87	63.2	48.5
Critical incident and trauma	98	56.1	49.9
Internet-based (online) counseling	38	42.1	50.0
Financial/legal	137	40.9	49.3
Work–life	96	33.3	47.4
Childcare/eldercare services	45	57.8	49.9
Expatriate support services	94	26.6	44.4
Concierge services	62	46.8	50.3
Coaching	167	35.3	47.9
Human Resource consultation	190	8.4	27.8
Performance management	168	7.7	26.8
Management training	170	47.1	50.1
Other specialist training (healthy lifestyle)	72	47.2	50.3
Stress management	66	54.5	50.2
Harassment, bullying, or grievance investigation	105	11.4	32.0
Workplace mediation	79	26.6	44.5

In Figure 6, the services are ranked from present in most companies toward present only in a small percentage of the companies. This graph shows that the majority of companies (between 80% and 60%) do have the more strictly HR-related services such as HR consultation, management training, performance management, and coaching. Almost one half of the

TABLE 3 Valid N, Mean Satisfaction Ratings (1–7), and Standard Deviation for the List of 18 Employee Services

Current status satisfaction	Valid N	M	SD
Counseling_depressive, panic, or anxiety	150	4.833	1.358
Counseling_stress & motivation	140	4.971	1.211
Alcohol & other drug	89	4.966	1.265
Critical incident and trauma	96	5.375	1.216
Internet-based (online) counseling	41	5.146	1.174
Financial/legal	136	5.015	1.282
Work–life	94	5.287	1.197
Childcare/eldercare services	48	5.167	1.449
Expatriate support services	92	5.130	1.141
Concierge services	65	5.246	1.199
Coaching	167	5.228	1.325
Human Resource consultation	201	4.930	1.377
Performance management	174	4.839	1.380
Management training	179	4.994	1.339
Other specialist training (healthy lifestyle)	73	5.192	1.151
Stress management	67	5.209	1.213
Harassment, bullying, or grievance investigation	106	5.113	1.132
Workplace mediation	80	5.125	1.216

Presence of the services

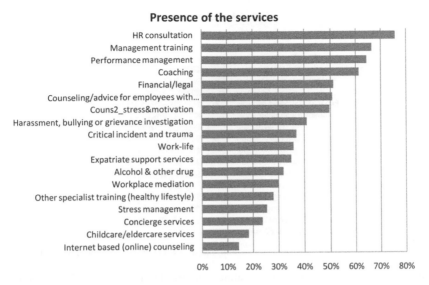

FIGURE 6 Percentage of companies that currently have the service available ranked from high to low.

companies seem to have the more typical EA services such as counseling and financial and legal advice available. A third group consists of critical incidents and trauma, work–life services, alcohol and drugs, and mediation. They are available in 40% to 30% of the companies. Finally, Internet-based services, stress management, other specialist trainings, concierge and childcare/eldercare services are available in less than 30% of the companies.

The previous data gave us an idea of whether these services are available, but it is important to be aware of the fact that this not mean that these services are delivered by an external EAP provider. The first group of services (HR-related services) in Figure 6 are typically taken up by internal channels, except for the management training (47% external). Counseling, alcohol and drug, critical incident, and trauma support are provided by external organizations in one half of the companies. Also stress management and childcare and eldercare are provided by external organization in more than 50% of the companies. Furthermore, it is striking that harassment investigation (11%), workplace mediation (27%), and work–life services (33%) are also mainly taking care of internally.

In Figure 7, the services are listed in function of their satisfaction scores. All the satisfaction scores were compared with each other using t tests for dependent samples. In general terms for this sample, it can be stated that a satisfaction difference score between two services is statistically meaningful when larger than 0.30 unless only a small group of respondents indicated the service was present in their company.

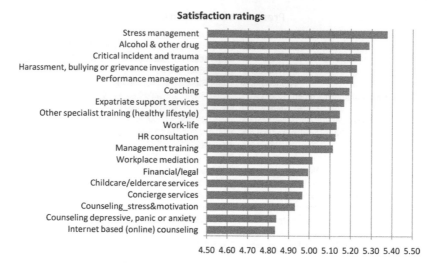

Satisfaction ratings

4.50 4.60 4.70 4.80 4.90 5.00 5.10 5.20 5.30 5.40 5.50

FIGURE 7 Satisfaction ratings on a 1–7 rating scale for the list of 18 employee services. The figure shows that the highest satisfaction scores are reached by stress management, alcohol & drug support, and critical incident and trauma services. The lowest satisfaction score is for the counseling services, concierge, and childcare/eldercare services.

Desired Status: List of Services

In Table 4 the mean scores of the usefulness/importance rating on a scale from 1 (*not at all*) to 7 (*very much*) are presented for all the services.

TABLE 4 Valid *N*, Mean Indicated Need (1–7), and Standard Deviation for the List of 18 Employee Services

Desired status	Valid *N*	Mean need (1–7)	*SD*
Counseling_depressive, panic, or anxiety	251	5.33	1.37
Counseling_stress & motivation	256	5.61	1.30
Alcohol & other drug	255	4.76	1.72
Critical incident and trauma	255	5.25	1.57
Internet-based (online) counseling	254	4.19	1.74
Financial/legal	252	5.05	1.45
Work–life	255	5.20	1.40
Childcare/eldercare services	255	5.04	1.62
Expatriate support services	252	4.52	1.80
Concierge services	250	3.78	1.66
Coaching	254	5.65	1.32
Human Resource consultation	253	5.76	1.30
Performance management	254	5.63	1.31
Management training	254	5.81	1.23
Other specialist training (healthy lifestyle)	254	4.59	1.54
Stress management	252	5.47	1.36
Harassment, bullying, or grievance investigation	254	5.30	1.65
Workplace mediation	252	4.83	1.63

TABLE 5 Valid *N*, Percentage Preferably External, and Standard Deviation for the List of 18 Employee Services

Desired status	Valid *N*	% External	*SD*
Counseling_depressive, panic, or anxiety	250	73.2	44.4
Counseling_stress & motivation	252	50.8	50.1
Alcohol & other drug	249	79.1	40.7
Critical incident and trauma	251	70.1	45.9
Internet based (online) counseling	242	65.3	47.7
Financial/legal	250	53.6	50.0
Work–life	248	49.2	50.1
Childcare/eldercare services	251	63.0	63.0
Expatriate support services	245	46.5	50.0
Concierge services	247	51.4	50.1
Coaching	252	43.7	49.7
Human Resource consultation	251	14.3	35.1
Performance management	249	18.9	39.2
Management training	250	48.0	48.0
Other specialist training (healthy lifestyle)	249	72.7	44.6
Stress management	247	61.9	48.7
Harassment, bullying, or grievance investigation	247	51.8	50.1
Workplace mediation	246	51.6	50.1

In Table 5 the proportion of respondents that would prefer to have an external person/organization responsible for this specific service is listed for all services.

When looking at Tables 4 and 5, the needs seem to be high for the HR-related services such as HR consultation, coaching, performance management, and management training (mean scores between 5.63 and 5.81 on the 1–7 scale). The needs are also high for counseling (5.61 and 5.23), critical incident support (5.25), work–life services (5.20), stress management (5.47), and harassment investigation (5.30). For concierge services, the need is the lowest (3.78) followed by Internet-based counseling (4.19).

Figure 8 below plots the different services in terms of their actual presence (horizontal axis) and their need (vertical axis). In the upper right panel the services are situated that score high in need and are present in the majority of the companies. In the upper left panel the services are situated that score high on the need-question but are not yet widely present in companies in Europe. In the lower left panel services are situated that are not widely present, but for which also the need is not very high. This figure gives a good idea of the services that have potential for growth and can take a larger market share in the future.

In Figure 9, the percentages of companies in which a specific service is actually delivered by an external provider are compared with the percentages for which it is desired that an external organization takes up the service. This gives us an idea of whether or not EAP companies are likely to sell these services to organizations. In general, there is a tendency for almost all services

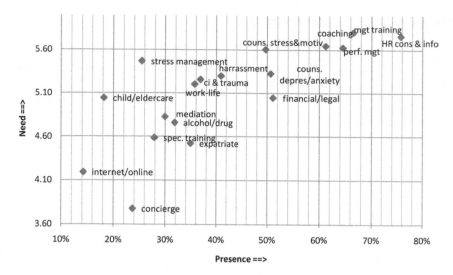

FIGURE 8 All 18 services plotted in function of their current percentage presence (0–1) and the indicated needs (1–7).

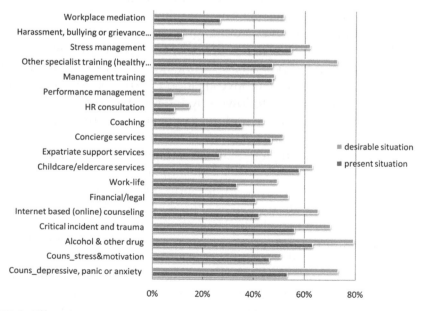

FIGURE 9 The percentage of companies in which the 18 employee services are currently provided by an external person or partner (dark bars) and the percentage of companies that would find an external partner useful (light bars). *Note.* HR = Human Resource.

TABLE 6 Valid *N*, Percentage Currently Present, and Percentage Desired for Each of the Different Aspects of Employee Assistance Services

Modus of delivery	Valid *N*	% Present	*SD*	Valid *N*	% Desired	*SD*
Website	262	53.1	50	254	85	35.7
Brochure	261	36.4	48.2	251	64.1	48.1
Individual counseling	259	54.1	49.9	255	80	40.1
Hotline	262	24	42.8	253	46.6	50
Online assessment + treatment	259	23.9	42.8	251	58.6	49.4
Family	259	20.5	40.4	251	53.4	50
Counseling by phone	257	63	63	244	63	63
E-mail	258	55	49.8	228	40.4	49.2
Chat	252	10.7	31	117	22.2	41.8
Training about communication and assertiveness	256	64.1	48.1	240	63.3	48.3
Work–life	254	32.7	47	238	60.1	49.1
Stress	254	48	48	246	48	48
Healthy lifestyle	249	31.3	46.5	118	24.6	43.2

to have them preferably provided by an external person/organization. Note that for management training the actual and the desired situation are close to each other. For counseling for depression/anxiety, workplace mediation, harassment investigation, and specialist trainings the gap between the actual and the desired situation seems to be the largest. Respondents would prefer to have these services external whereas they are mainly provided internally.

Different Aspects of EA Service Delivery

In Table 6 an overview is given for the questions about the modus of delivery of some of the services. Participants were asked to indicate to what extent the listed service was present and to what extent they considered such a service important or useful. The three graphs below give a visual overview of the discrepancy between the present situation and the desirable situation.

Figure 10 shows that the needs are high for information on websites and individual counseling or advice. These services indeed seem to be present in more than 50% of our sample. Also more than 55% would like to have

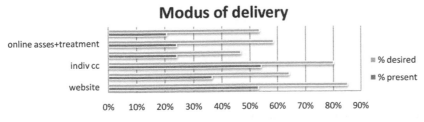

FIGURE 10 The percentage of companies that currently have these services available (% present, dark bars) compared to the percentage of companies that would like to have these services in place (% desired, light bars). *Note.* asses = assessment, indiv cc = individual counseling.

Contact with a counselor

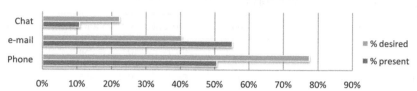

FIGURE 11 The percentage of companies that currently have counseling through chat, e-mail and phone (% present, dark bars) compared to the percentage of companies that would like to have these services in place (% desired, light bars).

information via brochures, online assessment and services for family members. These services are only available respectively in 36%, 24%, and 20% of the companies.

Although chat-services are only available in 10% of our sample (see Fig. 11), more than double of the respondents would like to have the possibility to chat with a counselor. E-mail communication is most often used but preference of our respondents clearly goes to phone communication.

The respondents of our sample indicate a clear need for trainings about stress, followed by work–life and communication skills as can be seen in Figure 12. Healthy lifestyle is considered less important (only 30% yes responses). In 60% of the companies communication training is available, in 40% trainings about stress and about 30% of the companies provides work–life and healthy lifestyle training.

Results for HR Managers

Table 7 shows the data of the questions filled in by the HR managers only. The percentage of the managers that currently uses an external organization or consultant for advice in the four different domains is presented as well as the extent to which the HR managers are satisfied with these services on a scale from 1 (*not at all*) to 7 (*very much*). The third part of Table 7 gives

Training

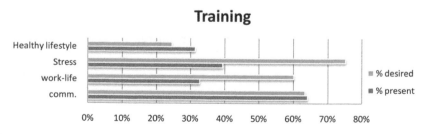

FIGURE 12 The percentage of companies that currently have training concerning healthy life-style, stress, work-life and communication and assertiveness available (% present, dark bars) compared to the percentage of companies that would like to have these services in place (% desired, light bars).

TABLE 7 Valid N, Percentage Currently Present, Mean Satisfaction Rating, and Percentage Desired with their Respective Standard Deviations for the Four Different Topics of Human Resource (HR) Advice

Advice for Human Resources	Valid N	% Present	SD	Valid N	Satisfaction	SD	Valid N	% Desired	SD
About communication/sensibilization?	68	63.2	48.6	42	5.238	0.878	57	56.1	50
About organizational surveys/audits?	67	59.7	49.4	39	5.103	1.188	57	56.1	50
About stress/health/well-being policy?	68	57.4	49.8	39	5.436	0.940	58	65.5	47.9
About action plans to improve well-being and health?	68	44.1	50	30	5.133	1.252	58	68.9	46.6

the valid N, mean, and standard deviation for the percentage of HR managers that find advice about these topics useful.

Table 7 makes clear that HR managers get advice about communication, surveys and audits, stress and well-being, but less about action plans about how to improve well-being and health. They are less satisfied about the advice for surveys and action plans and their need is the highest for action plans and well-being policy.

Comparison HR/Non-HR

In general the HR managers are more satisfied with the services than the workers as indicated in Figure 13.

With regard to their opinion about the need for specific services HR managers consider it more important than non-HR to provide counseling services, alcohol and drug support, critical incident and trauma support, HR consultation and information, performance management, management training and stress management services. In Figure 14, the differences in needs between HR and non-HR are presented.

With regard to the modus of delivery of the services HR managers give more importance to a 24/7 hotline, $t(251) = -2,67$, $p = 0.008$, and less to e-mail counseling, $t(229) = 2,26$, p 0.023, and training facilities in general, $t(244) = 2,06$, $p = 0.04$, than non-HR managers.

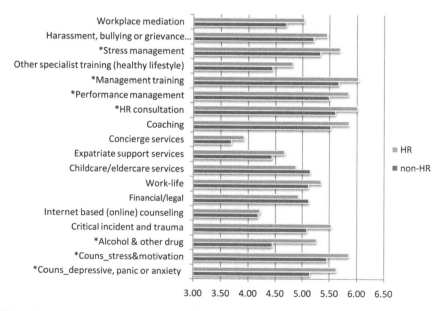

FIGURE 13 Satisfaction ratings on a 1–7 scale for each of the 18 employee services separately for Human Resource (HR, light blue bars) and non-HR (dark blue bars). *Services for which the needs indicated by HR and non-HR are significantly different on a $p < .05$ level.

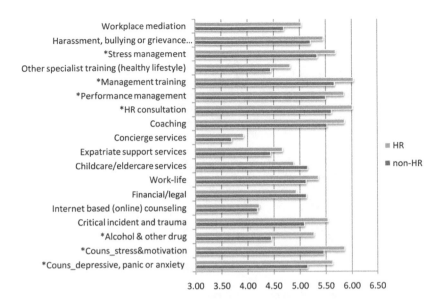

FIGURE 14 Needs on a 1–7 scale for each of the 18 employee services separately for Human Resource (HR; light bars) and non-HR (dark bars). *Services for which the needs indicated by HR and non-HR are significantly different on a $p < .05$ level.

Comparison Employees – Management

In comparison with the previous section where we made a distinction between employees and HR managers, for exploratory reasons we also divided our sample here in employees and management based on our question about staff category. The answers of those that have large responsibilities within companies (executives, management, and board: called management) on the one hand and employees (white- and blue-collar workers) on the other hand, were compared. We noticed that there was a group of persons in our non-HR that nevertheless had a very responsible function and therefore might have a different opinion on some of the issues under investigation.

In contrast with the above expectations however, this new division of our sample did not reveal any new insights as a very similar pattern of data was observed when a comparison was made between employees and management. Because no differences occurred, we found it not necessary to present this analysis in detail.

Comparison Between Countries

In Figures 15 and 16, the six European countries are compared respectively with regard to the presence of the different services and the perceived needs. In general, it becomes clear that the countries differ much more with regard to the presence of the services than with regard to the needs.

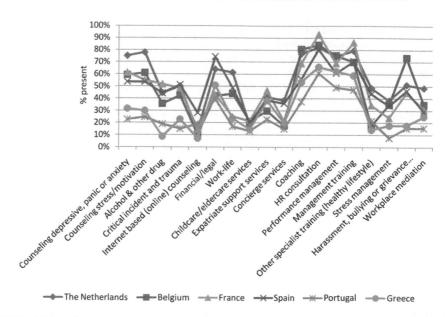

FIGURE 15 For the six countries separately, the percentage of companies that currently have each of the 18 services available is indicated. *Note.* HR = Human Resource.

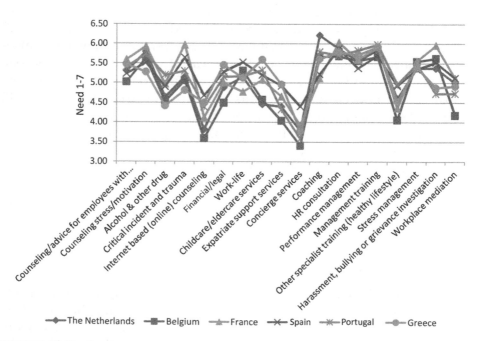

FIGURE 16 For the six countries separately, the mean indicated need (1–7) for each of the 18 services available is indicated. *Note.* HR = Human Resource.

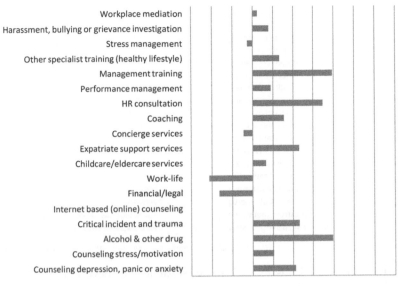

FIGURE 17 For France, for each service separately the deviation from the EU mean is indicated with regard to the percentage of companies in which this specific service is currently present. Positive scores indicate higher availability than the EU mean. Negative scores indicate lower availability. *Note.* HR = Human Resource.

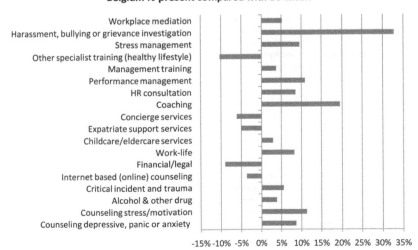

FIGURE 18 For Belgium, for each service separately the deviation from the EU mean is indicated with regard to the percentage of companies in which this specific service is currently present. Positive scores indicate higher availability than the EU mean. Negative scores indicate lower availability. *Note.* HR = Human Resource.

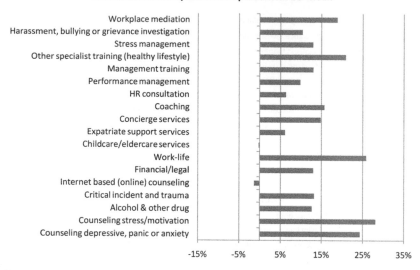

FIGURE 19 For the Netherlands, for each service separately the deviation from the EU mean is indicated with regard to the percentage of companies in which this specific service is currently present. Positive scores indicate higher availability than the EU mean. Negative scores indicate lower availability. *Note.* HR = Human Resource.

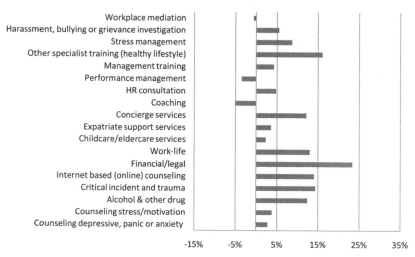

FIGURE 20 For Spain, for each service separately the deviation from the EU mean is indicated with regard to the percentage of companies in which this specific service is currently present. Positive scores indicate higher availability than the EU mean. Negative scores indicate lower availability. *Note.* HR = Human Resource.

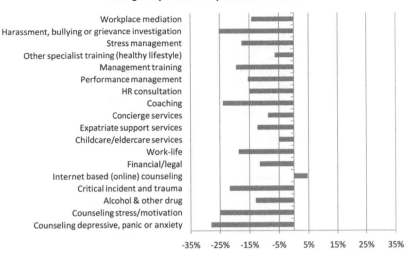

FIGURE 21 For Portugal, for each service separately the deviation from the EU mean is indicated with regard to the percentage of companies in which this specific service is currently present. Positive scores indicate higher availability than the EU mean. Negative scores indicate lower availability. *Note.* HR = Human Resource.

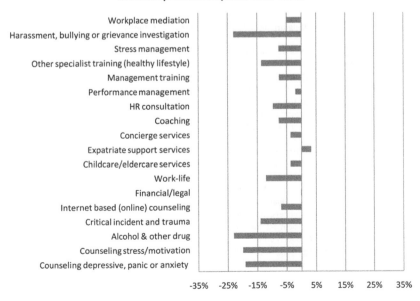

FIGURE 22 For Greece, for each service separately the deviation from the EU mean is indicated with regard to the percentage of companies in which this specific service is currently present. Positive scores indicate higher availability than the EU mean. Negative scores indicate lower availability. *Note.* HR = Human Resource.

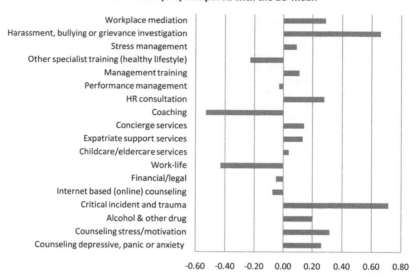

FIGURE 23 For France, for each service separately the deviation from the EU mean is indicated with regard to mean score on the need scale (1–7) for this specific service. Positive scores indicate higher needs than the EU mean. Negative scores indicate lower needs. *Note.* HR = Human Resource.

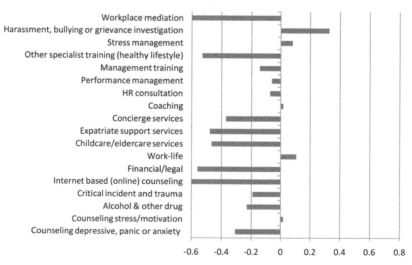

FIGURE 24 For Belgium, for each service separately the deviation from the EU mean is indicated with regard to the mean score on the need scale (1–7) for this specific service. Positive scores indicate higher needs than the EU mean. Negative scores indicate lower needs. *Note.* HR = Human Resource.

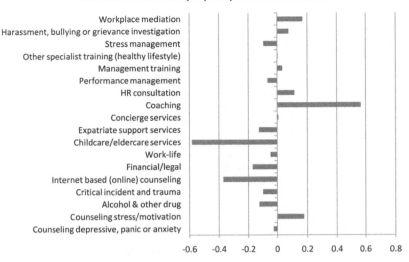

FIGURE 25 For the Netherlands, for each service separately the deviation from the EU mean is indicated with regard to the mean score on the need scale (1–7) for this specific service. Positive scores indicate higher needs than the EU mean. Negative scores indicate lower needs. *Note.* HR = Human Resource.

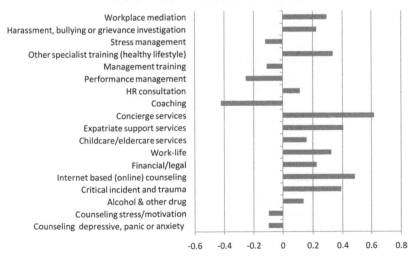

FIGURE 26 For Spain, for each service separately the deviation from the EU mean is indicated with regard to the mean score on the need scale (1–7) for this specific service. Positive scores indicate higher needs than the EU mean. Negative scores indicate lower needs. *Note.* HR = Human Resource.

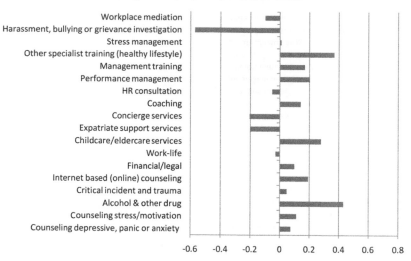

FIGURE 27 For Portugal, for each service separately the deviation from the EU mean is indicated with regard to the mean score on the need scale (1–7) for this specific service. Positive scores indicate higher needs than the EU mean. Negative scores indicate lower needs. *Note.* HR = Human Resource.

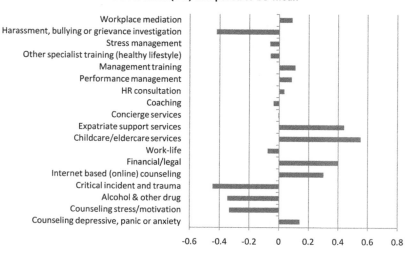

FIGURE 28 For Greece, for each service separately the deviation from the EU mean is indicated with regard to the mean score on the need scale (1–7) for this specific service. Positive scores indicate higher needs than the EU mean. Negative scores indicate lower needs. *Note.* HR = Human Resource.

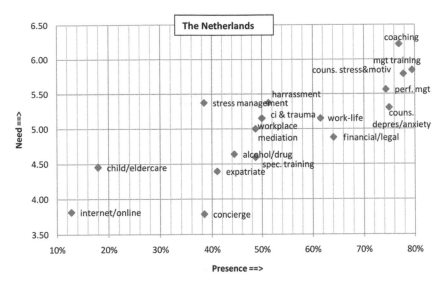

FIGURE 29 For the Netherlands, all 18 services plotted in function of their current percentage presence (0–1) and the indicated needs (1–7).

When looking at the services that are present, Portugal and Greece clearly have fewer services available and this seems to be the case for traditional EAP-related services as well as for more HR-related services. In The Netherlands most services are present in higher percentages than in other countries. Below for each country

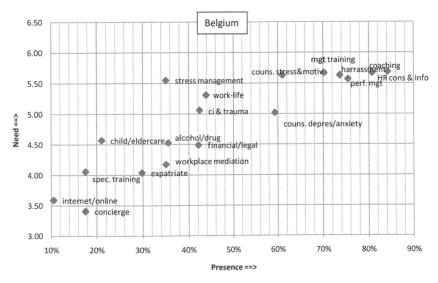

FIGURE 30 For Belgium, all 18 services plotted in function of their current percentage presence (0–1) and the indicated needs (1–7).

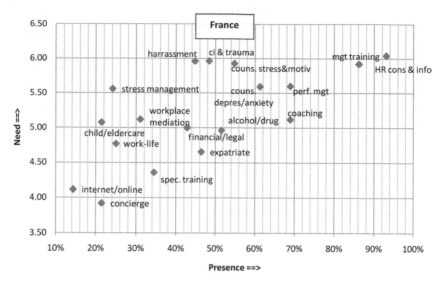

FIGURE 31 For France, all 18 services plotted in function of their current percentage presence (0–1) and the indicated needs (1–7).

a profile is presented, where the % present for each services is compared with the EU mean.

Although the needs are in general rather in line with each other (see Figure 16), different patterns are nevertheless occurring depending on the specific context in each country. In the figures (Figures 17–34) next, one can see what the needs are for each country compared to the EU mean.

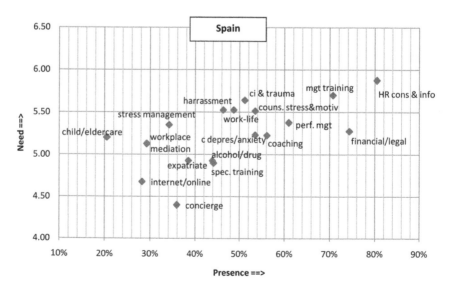

FIGURE 32 For Spain, all 18 services plotted in function of their current percentage presence (0–1) and the indicated needs (1–7).

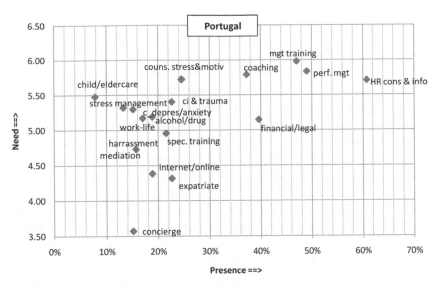

FIGURE 33 For Portugal, all 18 services plotted in function of their current percentage presence (0–1) and the indicated needs (1–7).

Finally, for each country also the needs are plotted against the present situation. In Figures 29–34 for each country, one can find the needs on the vertical axis and the presence on the horizontal axis.

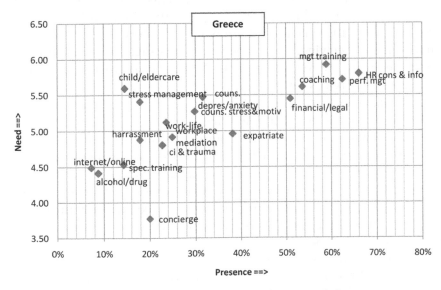

FIGURE 34 For Greece, all 18 services plotted in function of their current percentage presence (0–1) and the indicated needs (1–7).

GENERAL CONCLUSIONS

This study gives an important overview of the type of services that are currently available for companies in continental Europe. The HR-related services, that is, HR consultation and information, management training, performance management, and coaching are present in more than 60% of the companies. These services are mostly taken up internally except for management training where external partners are used in 47% of the cases. Satisfaction ratings are between 5.10 and 5.20 on a 1 to 7 scale situating these services in the middle range for satisfaction. The analysis also shows that these services are considered very useful (higher than 5.6 on the 1–7 need scale). Just like it is the case for most other services, our respondents would prefer slightly more than the present situation to have external help with these services. The one exception here is management training where the present and the desired situation already meet.

Counseling and advice for depression and anxiety and for stress and motivational problems seem to be present in 50% of the companies, receive rather low satisfaction scores and are taken up by an external provider in 50% of the cases. There is a clear need for these services and more often our respondents would like to have these services provided externally. So this seems to be an area with still some potential for growth. Also financial and legal advice is present in almost 50% of the companies, but the need is lower compared with the counseling services.

A third group of services are critical incident and trauma support, harassment, bullying, or grievance investigation and work–life services. They are present in 35% to 40% of the companies, the indicated need for these services is rather high, and they get rather high satisfaction scores. For these services there is also a high need for external delivery. Especially for harassment, bullying, and grievance investigation the services are currently taken up by internal persons (89%) but there is a clear need to outsource these services up to 52%.

Stress management seems to be a domain that clearly needs the attention of EAP providers in Europe as it has still a lot of potential for growth. It is yet only present in 30% of the companies and the indicated needs are high. Moreover the satisfaction with the services when available is also quite high and companies look for external organizations to supply the services.

Another service with a lot of potential is the child/eldercare service. Needs are high (above 5) and currently these services are only present in less than 20% of the companies. This is also typically a service that is outsourced by companies in Europe.

Alcohol and drugs support and workplace mediation are present in approximately 30% of the companies. Needs are relatively high and our respondents clearly indicate they want external support for these services. There might be good reasons for preferring an external provider for these services. As is also the case for harassment, bullying, and grievance investigation, anonymity and confidentiality can be much better covered by a neutral and therefore specialized external provider EA providers have good arguments to sell these services to companies and take over some of the services that are currently provided by internal partners.

The European market does not seem to be really ready yet for Internet-based (online) counseling. The need is currently low. However, when asking about the need for online assessment and treatment programs, 60% of the respondents indicated to find it useful and also when asking for the different ways of getting into contact with a counselor the option of using a chat service is indicated by more than 20% of the respondents, which is 10% more than the percentage of current availability. On the other hand, e-mail contact with a counselor is present in more than 50% of the companies and is clearly a less desired way of getting into contact. Although we need to be careful with this interpretation, these data might indicate that the need for personalized online services might grow in the future. Expatriate services are present in more than 30% of the companies and the need for them is moderate.

Finally, the specialist trainings are present in 28% of the companies and the need for these trainings seems to be moderate. When looking at our questions about the content of trainings, it becomes clear that there is more need for trainings about stress, work–life, and communications skills than there is for healthy lifestyle. It might be the case that the latter services are still considered more as "private" issues where actions of an employer are neither desirable nor convenient. With regard to the potential for growth looking at the difference between the present trainings available and the needs, stress, and work-life workshops seem to have the largest potential.

With regard to the modus of delivery some interesting findings are worth mentioning. Family services are currently not very common in Europe, but the reported usefulness of such services is rather high. These results seem to confirm the results of the child/eldercare services showing that in general this domain has future potential. Although individual counseling and coaching is present in more than 50% of the cases, hotlines are less popular. For both of these services there is still a clear gap between the desired and the present situation.

Our research was also specifically set up to make a comparison between the needs of HR managers and the needs of employees. In general, HR managers report that employee services are in general more available and of better quality than the end users of these services. It is not completely clear why that is the case but it is possible that information and communication about EA services toward the employees are playing a crucial role here. In many organizations services are available but very often employees are not very well informed about whom they will get into contact with, what they can expect, and so on. The results seem to suggest that this is an important area for improvement of the services. With regard to the needs, HR managers report higher needs than the employees for counseling services, alcohol and drug support, critical incident and trauma support, HR consultation and information, performance management, management training, and stress management and hotlines.

A final research goal was to illustrate the diversity in availability and embedding of EA services in the different countries in Europe. One important conclusion is that EA services are in general less present in Portugal and Greece than in the other four countries under investigation. Spain in contrast seems to be more comparable with France and Belgium, though coaching and performance management are less common in Spain. Also the high availability of financial and legal advice in Spain is striking and clearly different from Belgium and France where this service is less common. The Netherlands seems to have a large number of services available combined with an extremely high need for individual coaching. In Belgium most services seem to be present and the specific legal obligations that exist for companies with regard to well-being and harassment and bullying might explain the high score for harassment, bullying, or grievance investigation in Belgium. Also a very important observation is that in general the needs indicated by the specific countries are much less diverse than the availability of the services. France seems to indicate a higher need for critical incident and trauma support and harassment, bullying or grievance investigation, this might be related to some recent work-related "suicide" incidents with a lot of media attention.

This study did reveal important information for the EA field and can be considered as an important contribution and next step in the EAP research in continental Europe as well. Building further on the valuable findings of the Buon and Taylor (2007) study, we presented a list of EA services without assuming that all respondents are familiar with the concept of EAP nor putting forward a specific model or definition of what EAPs are. In comparison with the Buon and Taylor study, we managed to reach a much larger sample that also contained information about the employees' perception and not only from the perspective of the HR managers. Moreover, the collected data came from six different countries in Europe and also gives detailed information about the specific embedding of EA services in these countries.

Although we reached a rather large and diverse number of respondents for European norms, our sample is still rather small compared with the total amount of companies in Europe or compared with most data samples available in comparable studies in the United States. The collection of the present data took indeed a lot of effort and was more difficult than expected at first. A couple of factors might explain these difficulties. First, our questionnaire was rather long and repetitive. Second, the questionnaire was set up in English and for a lot of our potential respondents filling in a questionnaire in English asked some additional effort especially for employees in Spain and France. Third, we took the option to guarantee our respondents full anonymity to lower the threshold for participation in our research however this created also the practical difficulty that we were not able to see whether persons in fact filled in the questionnaire and therefore sending reminders was kept to a minimum. Fourth and last, we started our research without giving any incentive to our respondents, therefore we were not able anymore to change this condition toward the end of our data collection when we were in strong need for more respondents and would have considered to give an incentive for filling in the questionnaire.

Despite the rather small sample however, we have nevertheless reasons to believe in the robustness of our general findings. Halfway our research project, we did some preliminary analysis of the data and presented these data at the EAEF conference in Athens. Since then, we more than doubled the number of respondents and basically the same general conclusions came out of this analysis.

Another limitation is that our sample, though representative with regard to the criteria set up beforehand, might still be selective in the sense that we used our own broad network to collect the data. The respondents included might therefore be already more aware of, or interested in the general topic of mental health and psychosocial workplace issue. This will be particularly true for the HR managers involved in this study and hence some caution with the interpretation of our results is at stake. In general, however this would mean that the present data might contain an overestimation and that the actual presence of the services is lower than presented in the study. However the same might be considered true for the needs reported as HR managers already involved with these issues might score higher on the needs as well. For the employees of this sample, this drawback will probably play less as mainly personal and anonymous contacts through contacts of contacts are used to collect this part of the sample.

A third limitation is that we did not ask our respondents to indicate whether they have a formal EA service present in their company. This would have given us the opportunity to compare the needs of those that are not familiar with EAP and those who are. However, this limitation is a direct consequence of one of the main strengths and uniquenesses of this study namely starting with an open and nonbiased view on employee services regardless of the present globally and structurally present EAP market.

To conclude, this report reveals a lot of new information about the current as well as the future needs of employee services in continental Europe. It might be clear from this report that a lot of creativity and flexibility as well as an open mind with regard to cultural diversity will be necessary to let EA work flourish in continental Europe. Hopefully, this report will also help to put EA and mental health in general on the agenda of European policy makers. Future research might zoom into specific aspects or subareas of the EA business in Europe. For example, one area coming out of this study that needs more clarification is the online and Internet assessment, treatment, and counseling. Another route might be to broaden up the perspective and compare the tendencies in Continental Europe with tendencies in EA business in other regions in the world. One straightforward example is to use the present questionnaire and collect data in the United States, Australia, Asia, and Africa and compare their needs with the present needs and situation in continental Europe.

FUNDING

The study was funded by a grant from the Employee Assistance Research Foundation.

NOTES

1. These numbers are based on data made available through Eurostat (2009).
2. A copy of the full questionnaire as it was used in our study can be obtained by writing to the authors.
3. ISW Limits has built up a large benchmark with the Short-Inventory on stress and well-being (S-ISW) with data from more than 50,000 employees in Europe (mainly Belgium, France, and the Netherlands).
4. These numbers are based on data made available through Eurostat (2009).
5. These numbers are based on data made available through Eurostat (2009).

REFERENCES

Bhagat, R. S., Steverson, P. K., & Segovis, J. C. (2007). International and cultural variations in employee assistance programs: Implications for managerial health and effectiveness. *Journal of Management Studies, 44*, 222–242.

Buon, T., & Taylor, J. (2007). *A review of the employee assistance program market in the UK and continental Europe. Employee Assistance European Forum-EAP Study*. The Hague, the Netherlands: EAEF and Robert Gordon University.

Eurostat. (2009). *European business: Facts and figures*. Brussels, Belgium: Author.

Harnois, G., & Gabriel, P. (2000). *Mental health and work: Impact, issues and good practices*. Geneva, Switzerland: WHO and ILO.

Hopkins, R. (2005). The Employee Assistance European Forum (EAEF) and its role in the emerging EA market in continental Europe. In D. Masi (Ed.), *The International Employee Assistance Compendium* (3rd ed.; pp. 46–59). Boston, MA: Masi Research Consultants, Inc.

Reddy, M. (2005). The once and future EAP. In D. Masi (Ed.), *The International Employee Assistance Compendium* (3rd ed.; p. 3). Boston, MA: Masi Research Consultants, Inc.

Innovative Career Support Services for Professional Women in India: Pathways to Success

BEVERLY YOUNGER, PhD

University of Southern California School of Social Work, Los Angeles, California, USA

KALPANA TATAVARTI, MS, and NEETI POORSWANI, MSW

Interweave Consulting Pvt Ltd, Bangalore, India

DENICA GORDON-MANDEL, MSW, MA, BA,
CAITLIN HANNON, MSW, IKIAH K. MCGOWAN, MSW, BBA, and
GOKUL MANDAYAM, PhD

University of Southern California School of Social Work, Los Angeles, California, USA

This article examines the emerging concerns of professional working women in India, highlighting their unique needs within the context of rapidly changing environs and sociocultural gender expectations. An innovative intervention model that supports the goals of female professionals to sustain and succeed in their career, created by a women-managed consulting and training firm in Bangalore, India, is presented. An exploratory analysis of the impact of the group-based intervention modules, drawing upon detailed case studies and post-training surveys, is summarized. The qualitative analysis identified participants' outcomes using interview data from two availability samples: (a) case studies drawn from multiple multinational organizations (N= 16) and (b) case studies drawn from a single multinational organization (N= 12). Descriptive evaluation survey outcomes from a third organization sample (N= 71) were utilized. The identified themes included the evidenced adaptations of participants to work–life stressors, gender issues, and internal and organizational glass ceilings through their use of mentors, networking, assertiveness, and strategies for taking control of their career paths. The findings are relevant to advancing female career support services.

INTRODUCTION

Although Indian and transnational corporate organizations are realizing the contributions of the female workforce to India's economic growth, attitudes toward women workers and career support infrastructure for female talent have not kept pace. Women's labor participation rates are higher now than in the last century, yet this rate actually declined during the period of 2005 to 2010 (Lahoti, 2013), indicating a problem in female workforce sustainability.

Gender beliefs, internalized by women and their key stakeholders, affect their career choices and their ability to achieve work–life balance. This in turn results in the "leaking pipeline" of professional Indian women, with significant numbers of women dropping out before they reach the senior rungs of the organization ladder.

This study explores professional women's responses to innovative intervention model, Pathways to Success, created by a women-managed consulting and training firm in Bangalore, India, that supports the goals of female professionals to effectively climb the organizational ladder and to succeed in their careers.

LITERATURE REVIEW

Indian Professional Women in the Workforce: The Gender Gap and Glass Ceiling

From a historical perspective women in India are making relatively good gains in employment, improving their economic conditions, and finding independence and accomplishment (Budhwar, Saini, & Bhatnagar, 2005; Lahoti, 2013). The Society for Human Resource Management (2009) saw Indian women as an important, but not fully recognized, management talent pool and the increase in female managerial employment as a force for change in the status of women in India.

Yet India's gender gap remains wide, as defined by a set of economic and social indicators that include economic empowerment, education, marriage, maternity, and childcare trends, and social and political rights. India's gender gap is ranked 101 out of 136 countries in 2013 (Bekhouch, Hausmann, Tyson, & Zahidi, 2013). Indian women as a whole still face dense economic and social barriers when seeking to grow their careers.

Entering the workforce does not by itself guarantee an easy path to empowerment. Patriarchal culture, lingering gender stereotypes, differential treatment, and male egos challenge women who seek to become managers or to move upward in the organization (Budhwar et al., 2005; Haynes & Ghosh, 2012; Naqvi, 2011). Furthermore, traditional gender roles projected on women in the workplace often render women "invisible," requiring them to achieve more than men to be recognized (Patel & Parmentier, 2005).

Indian women, like many women globally, face economic and social glass ceilings, limiting women's progression toward promotion and management positions (Haynes & Ghosh, 2012). The ceiling is constructed of hard institutional realities, such as limited policies or policy enforcement, and management practices, as well as soft but durable sociocultural norms and behaviors.

Women encounter barriers such as the "maternal wall," a projection of limited competence for taking maternity leaves, and a "competence penalty," or perceptions of being too competent on the job (Williams, 2004, p. 17). These barriers may restrict the upward mobility of female professionals working in Indian-based corporations (Haynes & Ghosh, 2012). Global rates of women in senior management hover about 10%, but the rate lingers lower in India, with about 3% to 6% of women reaching senior levels (Budhwar et al., 2005). All of the above may diminish a woman's "career persistence," or the ability to avoid dropping out of the workforce regardless of marriage, motherhood, or other challenges (Srinivasan, Murty, & Nakra, 2013, p. 211).

Other organizational ceiling elements include the unique demands of specific industries or jobs required of professionals as they climb upward in the company's hierarchy. Men may be more able to work long hours, different shifts, or relocate more easily, whereas women may be more likely to say "if the need arises, then family comes first"(Valk & Srinivasan, 2011, p. 43).

On the positive side, women professionals are viewed as offering unique value to organizations, having more sensitive perceptions, better relationship awareness, a high commitment level, the ability to multitask, and a greater tendency to share power and seek input from others (Budhwar et al., 2005). Tarr-Whelan (2009) noted that women in senior positions have better fiscal outcomes (due to being more aware of risks, less reactive to losses), influence the advancement of policies that support health and education, further work–life integration and well-being, emphasize individual and corporate responsibility, and encourage participatory decision-making teamwork. Globally, businesses are welcoming the unique gifts that women bring to the workplace, and "a spike in demand" for female candidates is now being witnessed (Krishna, 2013, p. 18).

Familial and Social Influences on Women's Career Persistence and Success

Women's rapid movement into the workforce has put pressure on traditional familial roles in Indian homes. Luke and Munshi (2011) conceptualized an increase in women's income as challenging social norms, perceived by society as "weakening the family's ties to the ancestral community" (p. 16). In the same study, increased income was found to be associated with more household power for women and greater marital violence. In addition, family commitment and obligations are still a strong influence on female talent. In a study of professional Indian women, 84% agreed that "the female spouse was expected to take care of the family responsibilities," and 95% agreed that "commitment to family responsibility hindered the prospects of career advancement for women professionals" (Buddhapriya, 2009, p. 37).

Work and independent income are linked to some degree of autonomy and decision-making within families. The National Family Health Survey, 2005 to 2006, reveals factors associated with higher rates of women's decision-making power in Indian families. Older employed women, age 40 to 49, living in nuclear families in urban environments, with 12 or more years of education, and greater wealth, reported higher rates of decision-making power, either alone or in conjunction with their husband (International Institute for Population Sciences and Macro International, 2007, p. 464). Decisions over one's own health care, making major or daily household purchases, and visits to families and relatives are more easily made by women with greater social and economic power, allowing them more control over difficult work–life balance choices (International Institute for Population Sciences and Macro International, 2007).

The ability to balance dual roles appears to be related to familial life stages. One study found that 51% of women surveyed felt pressured to leave work upon getting married, and 52% at the time of childbirth (Hewlett, Rashid, Leader-Chivee, & Fredman, 2010). Claramma (2007) found that traditional family roles are more likely emphasized during the first two stages of a women's career stage model. A later stage may occur, called professional resurgence, during which one's maternal role needs decrease and career becomes the primary focus (Claramma, 2007).

It may be necessary to consider whether work–life balance is truly an achievable reality, or if some degree of stress and imbalance may continue to exist for women coping with dual roles. In a study of 180 married working women in Pondicherry, 82.2% of the sample perceived they were not able to achieve work–life balance (Delina & Raya, 2013, p. 278). Certainly a better understanding of women's unique career challenges will help to guide the development of successful career support services.

Work–Life Balance Factors

Work–life stressors may be culturally specific or even family specific. In India, cultural expectations in "joint families," or families with more than one generation cohabitating, deal with greater role expectations as they care for older family members and parents in law. Work–family balance includes dealing with family members' influence on a woman's personal choices, multiple role responsibilities and effectively negotiating these roles (Valk & Srinivasan, 2011).

The most intense stress is felt at the family and work intersection, where competing needs meet. In a 2011 study of 6,500 women in 21 countries, 87% of Indian women reported feeling time pressured, overworked and stressed, representing the highest stress levels of all women interviewed (Nielsen, 2011). In a study of 350 professional women in Kerala, lack of time, work overload, and home management pressures had the greatest negative impact on their work–life balance (Claramma, 2007). Women identified spousal support as the most important source in reducing dual role conflict, followed by the nature of the work, and the absence of young children. In Claramma's (2007) study, 81% stated that "the husbands do not look after the affairs of the family when they are busy at work" (p. 176).

A variety of other factors can complicate achieving work–life homeo-stasis, including the long commutes in urban areas, the persistent lack of available child care, limited domestic help in the home, or even managers who perceive flextime policies or benefits as being too difficult to implement (Desai, Majumdar, Chakraborty, & Ghosh, 2011).

For many professional women, the inability to balance dual roles can lead to negative outcomes. Seventy percent of women surveyed in Buddha-priya's (2009) study said that they worry about the effect of work stress on their health (p. 277). A study of married women in the information technology (IT) sector found that women who actually strive for work—life balance are more likely to have work stress and conflicts than women who strive less to achieve that balance (Appelbaum, Asham, & Argheyd, 2011). This implies that striving alone may not be the solution, and that some may surrender to the stressors by attempting to do it all, rather than attempting to set limits.

THE INTERNAL GLASS CEILING

The importance of affect and cognitive perceptions. The *internal glass ceiling* refers to a combination of emotional and cognitive perceptions that work in tandem with external realities to restrict working women's abilities to thrive in organizational environments (Ely, Ibarra, & Kolb, 2011). Caught in a work–life quandary, women professionals cope with an internal web of thoughts and emotions that may affect their ability to succeed in their careers.

Guilt is a significant emotion affecting women fulfilling the multiple roles of working women, wives, mothers, and daughters-in-law. Claramma (2007) believed they maintain internal guilt because of the strength of traditional role stereotypes, feeling the daily conflict of "who one is and what one should be doing" (p. 181). There is no official mechanism that counters the perception that traditional norms are being violated, even though acceptance of working women in India continues to grow.

In a study of women's career persistence, Srinivasan et al. (2013) utilized a career identity framework to explore the "attributes, beliefs, values, motives and experiences" that construct individuals' internalized identification with their career (p. 212). They discovered that career persistence increases when women score lower on a Beliefs about Gender Disadvantage (BGD) scale (a belief that gender bias exists. which in turn leads to disempowerment), and that career success was associated with career persistence (Srinivasan et al., 2013). Although lower BGD appears to be empowering, teaching women to ignore gender bias to gain a strong career identity and career persistence may be an oversimplification of workplace realities.

Lack of efficacy, or one's perceived ability to control one's environment, is another psychological state experienced by women attempting to balance what may feel unbalanceable. In a study of married working women, participants scored consistently high on the question, "I would like to reduce my working hours and stress levels, but feel I have no control over the current situation" (Delina & Raya, 2013, p. 277). A perceived lack of control was believed to be associated with a sense of powerlessness over one's environment. Boyar and Mosley's (2007) sophisticated model explored how internal self-evaluations may influence peoples' work–family outcomes among a sample of primarily married working women. They found that the higher one's core self-evaluation (which incorporates self-efficacy and self-esteem), the lower the participants' reported work-to-family conflicts.

The internal glass ceiling affecting women professionals in India has only begun to be explored. The assumption that strengthening women's self-efficacy will resolve their career needs, without first exploring the legitimacy of challenges women face upon entering the workforce, would be a travesty. Yet, using consciousness-raising techniques to realistically assess their situations, and dialogue and social support to alleviate guilt and blame, may more fully address their needs (Hossen, 2005).

Career Development and Support Services

Because female professional careers only began to be mainstreamed in the last century, organizations probably know as much about how to promote and develop women's career paths as the medical field once knew about women's health. To address this under-researched and newly established concern, human capital specialists and employers need to ask the question, "What is needed to effectively support women in their struggles against external and internal glass ceilings?"

The complex pressures affecting professional women are a recipe for job and career disengagement and stagnation, restricting women who could be moving upward and increasing their value to corporations. Jawahar and Hemmasi (2006) found a lack of organizational support for career advancement to be related to increased turnover intentions among professional women. In addition, they found that women professionals who perceive their employers as being supportive of their career are more likely to intend to stay in the job.

In Buddhapriya's (2009) study of professional women, a majority of those surveyed indicated that flexible working hours, child care facilities, and support for nonwork commitments would help them better achieve work–life balance. Work–life balance support may include standard flextime (part-time, tele-commuting, and job sharing) and innovative flextime (career break, parental and responsibility leaves) options that are becoming more commonly offered in businesses operating or located in India (Krishna, 2013).

Organizations may also choose to direct their efforts toward inclusion and career development actions. Gender diversity and inclusion initiatives for all female talent, and for C-suite and boardroom female executives, continue to trend as the value of female leaders becomes fully understood (Krishna, 2013). Career relaunch programs for women returning after maternity leaves or sabbaticals are becoming more common. Leadership development initiatives, supported by companies like IBM, seek to attract, bring back, sustain, and promote women leaders (Krishna, 2013). In a study of female Indian managers, 88% emphasized the need for career and leadership programs (Gupta, Koshal, & Koshal, 1998).

Haynes and Ghosh (2012) noted that supportive services such as "skill enhancement" and "women-only forums where women can construct social networks and build social capital within and across gender lines" are needed (p. 191). Gandhi (2013) called for businesses to identify women with strong potential early in their careers, followed by creating career development programs delivered by successful women managers. In addition, an inclusive organizational climate with open communication, and work–life balance accommodations are needed (Gandhi, 2013).

Yet, even with supportive environments, the responsibility to achieve balance will fall on the woman herself, who faces often a quagmire of difficult choices. Assertiveness development is recommended as a coping mechanism, including interventions aimed at increasing one's self-knowledge, practicing effective and honest communication with colleagues, exceeding expectations, matching the job to one's stage of career development, finding and using mentors for career guidance, and creating a goal-oriented career plan (Budhwar et al., 2005).

Work–life balance, employee assistance and wellness programs are potential sources of support, easing and addressing the effects of ongoing stressors. Buddhapriya (2009) found that 88% of professional women sampled agreed that Employee Assistance Programs for families with problems would be helpful, and 96% agreed that wellness and personal development programs would promote positive work–life balance (p. 39). Others advocate for special organizational centers to be developed where women workers learn to self-manage their needs, gaining skills such as "handling stress, relaxation, control of emotional and somatic responses, planning, problem solving, positive attitude and self-efficacy"(Desai et al., 2011, p. 444).

What is lacking is evidence related to the ability of innovative career support services to support women professionals as they navigate corporate waters, struggle to balance limited time and energy across dual roles, and strengthen their internal resources to sustain their career goals and increase their career persistence.

An Innovative Career Support Intervention

Interweave, a Bangalore-based diversity management consulting firm, developed Pathways to Success, a women-centric professional development program that addresses the internal glass ceiling and supports professional women's career success. This multitiered intervention applies an ecologically based model (Baral & Bhargava, 2010; Bronfenbrenner, 1986) focused on building a woman's capacity to cope with forces that hinder development of a professional identity and career success (Interweave Consulting Pvt Ltd, personnel communications, January 4, 2013).

Empowering Indian women to actively engage in career development requires a dynamic and broad approach. Interweave's approach focuses on (a) women in the context of their environment, (b) the centrality of work as a life activity, (c) how the role of work relates to family and societal roles, (d) the nonlinear career path of many women, (e) developing and managing career opportunities, and (f) managing the time demands of maintaining multiple roles. Pathways to Success modules were designed to foster a woman's sense of personal control at the interpersonal and professional level. The stated objective after completion of the program is for participants to have the mind-set and skills needed to progress in their professional life (Interweave Consulting Pvt Ltd, personnel communications, January 4, 2013).

After performing an organizational needs assessment, Interweave consultants collaboratively match Pathways to Success modules with client organizations to address the complexities of being an Indian woman working in that sector. Interventions are conducted in an all-female group format with participants identified and screened by the organization's human resources department.

Program modules stimulate and challenge women by "shedding light on internalized beliefs," then working to resolve conflicts between the woman, her professional identity, and the social structures that influence her decision making (Interweave Consulting Pvt Ltd, personnel communications, January 4, 2013). Interweave's 12 training modules are described below (see Table 1). The first four modules set the foundation for change, requiring introspection and reflection by group participants (Interweave Consulting Pvt Ltd, personnel communications, January 4, 2013). Programming examines social

TABLE 1 Intervention Modules and Intended Outcomes

Module	Intended outcomes for participants
Taking Charge	Taking responsibility for one's own growth
Positively Charged	Operating with an assertive style
Through the Looking Glass	Building a powerful brand and presence
Six Degrees of Relationship	Networking for success
A Cut Above	Commanding an executive presence
Influencing Upward	Influencing decision makers for career success
Power and the Woman	Expressing and exercising power for leading effectively
Yin and Yang	Embracing feminine and masculine behaviors for a holistic leadership style
Work-Life Synergy	Effectively combining various life pursuits
Win-Win	Negotiating for success
The Emotional Advantage	Making emotional intelligence work for you
Mentoring the Mentor	Up skill mentors and mentees for an effective mentoring relationship

norms that impact professional development, a woman's relationship with power and influence, work–life balance issues, as well as the importance of cultivating both professional and personal resources.

The consultants employ skill-building methodologies, such as situational analysis, and incorporate videos and role plays, action plan development, guided skills practice, and facilitator-participant feedback. Interventions are action-based, modeling behaviors and decision-making skills that allow the women to gain personal insight and understanding through transformational experiences. And, the women themselves are viewed as a valuable resource for their own professional development and for the professional development of other women, as well as being contributors within their communities.

METHOD

This explorative study presents findings from an analysis of detailed qualitative case studies and postworkshop evaluation feedback survey data, exploring participants' reactions to the Pathways to Success modules, among three samples of female professionals employed in different organizations in various locations across India. Available data collected and provided by the consulting firm's evaluation processes was utilized and analyzed by a team of researchers from a U.S.-based university.

Samples

The consulting firm's evaluation data was drawn from three separate samples (described below) of women professionals who had participated in one or more workshops over the last 2 years.

1. Multiple multinational organizations (MMO) case studies: This sample consisted of an availability sample of 16 female professionals working across several multinational organizations operating in India, from various professional sectors, including information technology, financial services, human resources, and retail. Participants attended one or more of a range of workshops as described above.
2. Single multinational organization (SMO) case studies: This sample consisted of an availability sample of 12 working women from various settings within a single multinational organization's worksites located across India. Participants attended one or more of range of workshops.
3. SMO Employees Evaluation Feedback Survey sample: This sample consisted of 71 female professionals, working in various settings of the same large, multinational organization from which the SMO case studies were drawn. The sample consists of participants who completed an evaluation feedback survey after attending one of the following Pathways to Success modules:
   - Power and the Woman ($N = 22$)
   - Influencing Upward ($N = 20$)
   - Six Degrees of Relationship ($N = 29$)

Data Collection Methods and Measurements

Data for the study was gathered by the diversity management consulting firm and provided to the researchers for purposes of analysis and interpretation of findings.

CASE STUDY DATA COLLECTION

The data collection method used with case study samples (MMO and SMO) consisted of semistructured in-depth interviews with participants who had attended one or more of the Pathways to Success modules. Participants' post-participation study contact times ranged from zero months to more than 12 months. Participant invitation was purposive only to the extent to which they represented a variety of locales and workshop types, but sampling was not specific to participants' demographics.

The interviewers, who were representatives of the consulting firm, used a semistructured interview schedule, with follow-up probes that varied by interview across participants, allowing fluidity for full exploration of emerging stories. The interview schedules for the two case study samples differed slightly. The MMO interview questions explored abilities and preparedness to achieve career goals, based on relevant external knowledge (ability to identify career opportunities) and internal knowledge (understanding of internal strengths), as well as changes in participants' career perceptions and behaviors on the job. The SMO interview questions, in addition to the areas covered by the MMO interview schedule, additionally inquired about career challenges, and organizational actions that would best support participants, as well as questions regarding their recommendations for content and delivery of future workshops.

The interviews were recorded, with participant approval, and audio files were used to make written transcriptions, which were then provided to the researchers for purposes of analysis. No identifying information was included with the data transcripts. Interviewees were not identifiable by the employer organizations or the research team, ensuring participants' rights to privacy of information, anonymity and confidentiality. Informed consent from the participants was obtained by the interviewers.

EVALUATION FEEDBACK SURVEY

A standard evaluation feedback survey routinely used by the consulting firm provided a source of existing descriptive data. The Course Evaluation Form consisted of nine quantitative questions, with a response set of 1 (*strongly disagree*) to 6 (*strongly agree*), which addressed the following areas:

- Facilitator knowledge, preparedness, and organization
- Courseware materials and usefulness on the job
- Learning effectiveness of training relative to knowledge and skills
- Applications of training knowledge and skills to job and job performance
- Overall course rating and facilitator effectiveness.

No identifying information and no demographic information were collected with the evaluation feedback survey, protecting participants' privacy of information, anonymity, and confidentiality.

An important limitation regarding the survey instrument is that it serves as a standard industry training feedback tool, and its reliability and validity have not been tested, and provided postintervention, exploratory level information only.

Data Analysis

CASE STUDY QUALITATIVE DATA ANALYSIS

Interview data were manually analyzed using written transcript databases organized by interview question across each participant. Using general qualitative research analysis methods, the researchers used coding to identify the initial level of themes. Connections across themes were identified to create a second level of concepts, and were organized into broader categories, which were framed by the themes inherent in the initial interview questions.

The broader categories were found to be largely consistent across the two case study samples (see Results), allowing results from the two samples to be combined into a single conceptual framework of the third-level categories. A manual analysis was used to fully engage with and retain the full context of the participants' responses.

EVALUATION FEEDBACK SURVEY ANALYSIS

The postintervention feedback survey data was analyzed by the use of mean scores and percentages of agreement relative to the sample size, providing descriptive findings to support the qualitative analyses.

RESULTS

Demographic Description of the MMO Sample

The sample comprised a total of 16 working women age 28 to 49 years, crossing various professional sectors (i.e., information technology, financial services, human resources, retail).

All participants held a postgraduate education. Marital and family status of the sample ranged from single women living with parents, to married women with children living cojointly with extended family, and married women with children living within a nuclear family.

Demographic Description of the SMO Sample

The SMO interview participants consisted of 12 working women from various organizations across a variety of locations in India. One half of the employees in the sample had worked for the organization for 10 or more years, two women for 5 to 10 years, and four women had worked fewer than 5 years within the SMO. Four of the women had not worked for any employer other than the SMO.

Personal demographics were only minimally explored by the SMO interviewer. In this sample, nine of the participants were married, six had a single child, and the remainder of six participants had no children. The participants were distributed across four different Indian states. Age, ethnicity or other information was not available.

Emerging Theme Categories and Selection

The highly specific purpose and focus of the interview process led to the creation of clear overarching categories, with resulting themes identified within these categories. The following categories stem partially from the initial goals for this study, as influenced by categories of semistructured interview questions:

- Challenges: Participants' career and work–life difficulties
- Changes: Participants' observations of differences after workshop participation
- General statements of the perceived value of interventions
- Helpful intervention techniques.

Within the Challenges and Changes categories, some resulting themes mirror content found in Pathways to Success modules, whereas other themes were unique to participants' current realities, as evidenced by common response patterns across participants. Themes, their definitions, and quotes from actual participants' statements are provided within each category, with examples from either the MMO and SMO or both samples. The large majority of participants' quotations are exact transcriptions with very slight modifications when needed for legibility.

Challenges: Participants' Career and Work–Life Difficulties

The Pathways to Success modules sought to increase women's awareness of the challenges they face in the workplace, fostering their ability to establish support systems that aide in professional development.

GENDER ROLES AND RELATED SOCIAL NORMS CHALLENGES

This emerging theme focused on participants' challenges triggered by social norms related to gender. These are the socially learned roles and behaviors that are often based on our gender identity (Patel & Parmentier, 2005).
SMO Example:

> I feel that women have to put a little bit more in their (job) interviews or wherever. It has to be a distinct proving before you get the job... somewhere you have to prove that you are little bit more than a man.

CHILD CARE LIMITATIONS CHALLENGES

Limitations of child care resources were discussed by participants in the MMO sample, but not in the SMO sample, which may have been due to a difference in available resources. Access to child care has been found to be significantly associated with employee retention within a large sample from Indian businesses (Babu & Raj, 2013).
MMO Example:

> I think that this is one of the biggest challenges, because apart from our social tradition ... of women being wives, mothers and employees ... India does not have a very good system in terms of, you know, if you are a working mother, who is there to take care of your child.

ASSERTIVENESS AND SELF-DEVELOPMENT CHALLENGES

Some participants spoke about their inner challenges in making change, identifying the aspects of themselves that were difficult to change. As the workshops stress the need for assertiveness and self-development, some women have to first confront their own internal self-motivation in order to succeed (Budhwar et al., 2005).

MMO Example:

> Of course, nowadays not many people are so confident to go up to a person and start speaking with them unless you really have a topic to discuss. You keep yourself so reserved and so isolated from the rest of the world and you keep thinking...just get up and ask that question. [But] I might be questioned back again, so I do have to have the answer ready with those questions all hovering around your mind. You end up not speaking at all, which keeps you all inside yourself.

RELOCATION CHALLENGES

Upward mobility often depends upon the flexibility to relocate to ascend the organizational chart. Current research indicates there is a tendency for married women to be perceived as lacking flexibility to relocate and therefore facing promotion limits (Nath, 2000).

SMO Example:

> The senior roles within the organization have localized in Mumbai, and postmarriage immobility unfortunately is a reality, which is the set of most married women.

ORGANIZATIONAL SUPPORT CHALLENGES

Although organizations make the effort to be inclusive and flexible to support work—life balance, as one participant reflected below, policies alone may not change attitudes. Yet, organizational support, such as work—life flextime, directly influences employees' attitudes toward the organization (Baral & Bhargava, 2010).

SMO Example:

> Even if the company puts rules in place, there are mindsets that need to change, and the mindsets need to change at the ground level, not necessary to be just at the senior management level, because at every recruitment process, the senior managers don't sit in for interviews. I am not saying they don't include women or there is a distinct bias, I wouldn't say that, otherwise I wouldn't be here for 25 years. But, I think somewhere they feel comfortable that women in this kind of a role is good, and cannot manage a different kind of a role.

Organizational Mentor Challenges

A lack of mentoring is considered one of the barriers to career advancement for women professionals (Buddhapriya, 2009).
MMO Example:

> [Have you been able to identify any mentors?] Not within my organization yet to be honest. But I definitely have a few mentors within the profession that I worked with. When I don't know someone too well, I do hesitate in reaching out. Because you really kind of wonder what the person is really going to think? Is it going to look like a complaint session? You kind of have all these different things going on in your head.

Changes: Participants' Observations of Differences after Workshop Participation

The majority of participants identified changes they had implemented, specific to the themes addressed in the workshops. The following themes include specific types of changes associated with workshop participation that were highlighted by the participants.

Identifying Gender Issues

A variety of opinions were expressed about the inclusion of women in the workplace, as interview questions focused on participants' awareness of gender issues after participating, and even whether men should be involved in workshops to further open the dialogue. Dialogue on discrimination and gender issues is an important element of conscious-raising (Hossen, 2005).
SMO Example:

> If we have to critically evaluate it, then sometimes the whole workshop was making people aware of harassment laws and things that should not happen. It is good to educate them and tell them that these are the statutory things that they should be aware of.

Managing Emotions

Guilt was a common focus for participants, and is also noted to be a reaction to failing to truly balance multiple, socially expected roles (Claramma, 2007). The Pathway to Success modules emphasized managing not only one's own and others' perceptions, but also one's own emotions.
MMO Example:

> Sometimes you think that you're the only woman feeling or experiencing the guilt factor or balancing issue. You definitely know that it's tough for all women who are playing the multiple roles and want to do everything

perfectly. But, this was a forum where people kind of brought in their views, shared some ideas and definitely helped you to learn how to deal with the situations when you come across them.

ASSERTIVENESS, SELF-KNOWLEDGE, AND STRENGTHS IDENTIFICATION

Participants tended to easily identify changes in their level of self-knowledge, assertiveness and strengths overall. Many commented on being more conscious of their strengths and ability to show strengths. Srinivasan et al. (2013) referred to women's career success being related to their career centrality or the sense that one's career is necessary and a core part of their social identity.
MMO Examples:

> I feel that I have understood that I am a lot more approachable and people find me to be very amicable, and right now I am comfortable in sharing my knowledge, my experience and not holding back with respect to something. In terms of assertiveness, yes, I need to develop some more of that. Otherwise, my strengths are I feel myself to be somebody who is very committed, and I definitely try to give 100% when I take up the responsibility or ownership of something. So people can count on me.

WORK–LIFE BALANCE ADAPTATIONS

Participants noted adaptations that they have made to gain a better work—life balance, some of which includes thinking about how to manage the work—life conflicts, as well as making gradual changes over time. Women with an internal sense of efficacy in achieving a work-life balance may be more likely to accomplish a better work-life balance (Boyar & Mosley, 2007).
MMO Example:

> How much? In percentage I would say about 70% out of 100. Why? Because that is again a juggling that is going on again right now, and I am struggling to keep both my work-life balance intact, so that nothing falls apart. So there is again a kind of a fight that goes on everyday of me trying to juggle things so stress is more on me rather than the surrounding parties, because if I am taking all of the juggling myself, then of course we have to manage everything else. So. sometimes you have to adjust to those situations or compromise or sometimes you get to the next level and you think "Ok let me take this challenge" and I will try to overcome the rest.

USING RESOURCES AT HOME

Practical and emotional support at home from one's family has work-related consequences, including reducing workplace stress (Wayne, Randel, &

Stevens, 2006). The workshop modules emphasized the importance of asserting one's need for support at home.

MMO Example:

> If you're outsourcing stuff like your household work, your daily house-hold, even the cooking you're outsourcing it, you should not feel guilty about it.

USING RESOURCES AT WORK

Requesting support and assistance at work is addressed in the workshops, requiring participants to increase their assertiveness and knowledge of available resources. A supportive environment, with manager and coworker support, can help female employees achieve a better work-life balance (Baral & Bhargava, 2010), but utilization of that supports requires women to be empowered to request it.

SMO Example:

> [Has your work organization been supportive of your career?] Yes certainly, they have been very supportive, in fact I am in a service role, I have an inclination towards sales, but I am not really comfortable in doing the outright sales job. They have been very supportive in giving that opportunity if I wanted to move on that, or nominating me for courses, which will help me on developing those skills. Whenever I have requested for any kind of training in terms of skill and knowledge development, they have assisted me with that.

BRANDING COMPREHENSION AND USE

Budhwar et al. (2005) discussed the importance of replacing stereotypes of women, as they are perceived in the workplace, with the unique strengths they evidence within organizations. This requires a re-branding, which is emphasized in the Pathway to Success module. Women tended to react positively to the idea of creating a personal brand for themselves.

SMO Example:

> We do have some Senior Management introducing the other global heads of our department coming to India, and a few of us were invited to have lunch with him and create ideas and to get his views. So, typically with senior management, you possibly, on a one-one basis, may have just 10–15 minutes. You have got to maximize an inch, and whatever say, you want to say in a most concise and effective manner. So after that workshop, my takeaway was to be better prepared and, you know, think it through as to how would I like to introduce myself, the key identities and ideas.

NETWORKING SKILLS AND USE

Understanding the importance of networking in today's business environment, and learning the skills of networking, were discussed by several of the participants. Some noted feeling uncomfortable at first with the process, but began practicing it more routinely after workshop participation. Naqvi (2011) indicated that women who are not able to network may fail to make progress and gain mobility in their careers.

MMO Example:

> I thought that I am a social person but professional networking is something that I used to struggle with. What would you really talk about it? I think I didn't know how important it is now. There is no other way to go but to build your professional network. So, another thing that I have really done is, though I was on Linkedin, I really didn't get myself connected to too many people that I know. So, I consciously try and do that now. Every weekend at least for a couple of minutes, I try and build my network, talk to people and see what they are doing in their own careers and exchange a few notes. So, I have been consciously doing that.

Mentoring use. Some participants have become actively involved in working with mentors, especially mentors within their organization, after participating in the program. Mentoring programs have shown success in supporting women in their career development paths (Dworkin, Maurer, & Schipani, 2012).

MMO Example:

> I speak to my mentor very regularly. She has always given me very candid feedback. We share a very open relationship when it comes to sharing feedback and I make sure that I go back to her and work on things. Last time, she told me that I display my emotions openly, which is not good. I don't necessarily contribute to meetings. So, that is something I have worked on and I have started contributing to meetings. I also have a few people that I mentor so I actually pass this on to them as well.

Social support and use. Haynes and Ghosh (2012) emphasized the importance of psychosocial support for Indian women entering or sustaining their careers as they struggle with cultural and organizational expectations. Some participants found that the workshops created new internal networks, and allowed for immediate, and in some cases, ongoing social support.

SMO Example:

> One of the good things about the workshop was we got together, and the more we share it in the group then we feel that you are in the community. Some of these things, which were always subconsciously going in your mind, where you will be persuading it, and whether you'll be selected

or not, and things like that. I think that the realization for me was quite critical; and getting together with women and other like-minded people helped me open up about some of these issues.

Career goals and planning. Several participants discussed implementing their own career planning and goal development process, within the context of the organization, or finding a way to integrate their goals with the organization's goals. Career planning is a significant component of an effective career strategy (Tan & Yahya, 2013).

MMO Example:

In reality, we have to think what we want to be in the next 10 years, and all those things. So, a planning kind of thing, which was not there much before attending the programme, has now changed . . . like what we want to be exactly. Overall, I know what I should be in the future, what should I achieve, and what is the organization's needs. And accordingly align the organizational goals with our goals. We have to go forward. In view of the next 10 years, somehow manage to prepare the goals and also to plan for the next 5 to 10 years. Along with goals, where we have to be . . . what we have to be . . . those kind of inputs were good.

Improvements on the job. A variety of participants noted specific changes that occurred on the job, at some point after participating in a workshop.

SMO Example:

So I feel that I have been able to implement it [program recommendations], and the kind of feedback that I got from my boss was positive, like how the people around me think, and how the colleagues are sharing how they are comfortable, and why I'm able to do what I have done. So to that extent, my boss has given pretty good feedback.

General Statements of the Perceived Value of Interventions

The following provide an example of participants' comprehensive statements about the overall value of participation in one or more workshops.

SMO Example:

I was thinking that it is okay [organization] has started an initiative, and it is good that [organization] is going to encourage women employment and giving them opportunities, and given areas where they can add value in terms of personal growth and things like that. Initially, I had to decline [attending] a little bit because of the work and the commitments that I had in my workplace. But later on I realized that it is very important to attend this workshop and understand how it is going to help me. Certainly it was good, the initial way of understanding the concepts and explaining the way how women can be different, and the power of women can be used in a positive way. It is something I liked.

MMO Example:

I think it [the program] just hit the right chord within us and will go a long way in helping women get to what they are aspiring for, and helping them actually get there because there are things that are needed, the support structure is very important for a woman to actually achieve their aspirations.

Helpful Intervention Techniques

When questioned about what aspects of the intervention module(s) were most helpful to them, participants indicated that role-playing, social support and sharing, getting to know their peers, and the use of guest speakers telling their career stories were helpful techniques used in the modules.

SMO Module Evaluation Feedback Survey Responses

A sample of 71 participants completed evaluation feedback forms after completion of a Pathways to Success module. All of the participants were female employees of the SMO. No demographic information was collected. The original purpose for this survey was to obtain participants' feedback on the workshop experiences, using a commonly used training feedback survey format, with nine Likert-type scale questions, using the anchored scale of 6 (*strongly agree*) to 1 (*strongly disagree*) with N/A (*not applicable*).

All of the ratings were strongly positive across all questions, from the module's ability to improve their job performance ($x = 4.7/6.0$), to the facilitator's knowledge level ($x = 5.4/6.0$).

The percentage of moderate to high agreement (ratings of 4, 5, and 6 on the response scale) was over 90% on all survey questions. When selecting only high agreement scores (5 and 6 on the Likert-type scale), all participants continued to demonstrate at least 77% agreement on all questions.

Participants' ratings of the Courseware and Job Impact questions were slightly lower, a finding greatly limited by the study design and simple descriptive statistics, but perhaps valuable to explore in a future evaluation (see Table 2).

DISCUSSION

The impact of gender roles in the workplace is established firmly in the literature (Budhwar et al., 2005) and was confirmed in the qualitative responses.

TABLE 2 Results of Evaluation Feedback Survey Responses

Categories of questions and actual questions $N=71$	Mean score scale: 1 to 6	Percentage of high agreement scores: 5 & 6	Percentage of moderate to high agreement scores: 4, 5 & 6
Facilitator			
The facilitator was knowledgeable about the subject	5.4	92	97
The facilitator was prepared and organized for the class	5.3	89	97
The facilitator's energy and enthusiasm kept the participants actively engaged	5.1	77	93
Courseware			
The participant materials (manual, presentation handouts, etc.) will be useful on the job	4.7	65	92
Learning Effectiveness			
I have learned new knowledge/skills from this training	4.9	77	96
Job Impact			
I will be able to apply the knowledge and skills learned in this class to my job	4.9	72	96
This training will improve my job performance	4.7	64	93
Overall Rating			
The course	4.9	75	93
The effectiveness of the facilitator	5.2	82	92

Women identified that they "have to prove that you are a little bit more than the men," while balancing intense career requirements with traditional pressures to perform their roles as wives, mothers, and family members. Participants reflected on the gender role guilt factor, and felt able to "help each other along the way." This process was reminiscent of consciousness-raising empowerment techniques used to increase women's awareness of gender struggles (Hossen, 2005).

Participant's challenges included the internal, emotional, and psychological glass ceiling, which for one participant was highlighted by her struggle to assert her needs and to "just get up and ask that question." Women professionals, responding to gender-role expectations, often struggle to secure and assert their career identity in a way that propels them to success (Patel & Parmentier, 2005). Yet, in response to interviewers' questions, participants referred to increased abilities to manage emotions, to assert themselves, and to identify their strengths.

Gaining awareness of cognitive and emotional challenges from which the internal glass ceiling is constructed frees female professionals to create well defined and visible career identities (Srinivasan et al., 2013). Learning to "maximize an inch," and "say what you want to say in a concise and effective manner," participants used workshop techniques to create their own brand that they will be remembered for. Integrating this into their work inter-actions is likely to reduce the risk of invisibility in business settings (Patel & Parmentier, 2005).

Women acknowledged their work–life balance struggles, and the reality that mothers continue to be the primary person dedicated to be responsible for knowing "who is there to take care of your child." The work-life adjustments require "struggling," "fighting," and "juggling" to meet chal-lenges. The emphasis on assertiveness in the workshops may be beneficial in empowering women to ask for needed support and resources.

Asking for career guidance is also a psychological and practical chal-lenge for professional women, with one participant noting that "I do hesitate in reaching out." Some participants identified the lack of internal mentors in their organizations. Overall, participants often described that they are now seeking out and working with mentors to guide their career paths. Embracing mentoring is likely to also increase their career success (Bozionelos, Bozionelos, Kostopoulos, & Polychroniou, 2011).

A useful effect of the workshops noted in several comments included the tendency for those attending workgroups to become a type of informal social support group within their organizations after participating. This created a "community" of "like-minded people," who were more likely to relate effectively to each other.

Networking was increased, as participants understood the need to "consciously try...and build my network." They also grasped the impor-tance of building and using networks over time, a crucial tool in career building for women (Naqvi, 2011).

Participants also clearly grasped the importance of strategically building their careers, through career planning and goal setting. One challenge noted among some of the participants was the lack of flexibility to relocate or to be mobile across organizational locations. The centralization of senior roles within the organization to a specific locale is part of the external glass ceiling for women, and "postmarriage immobility unfortunately is a reality." Career planning requires them to adapt to these promotion limitations (Nath, 2000).

Ultimately, employers see the value that professional women bring to the workplace (Budhwar et al., 2005; Krishna, 2013), and have engaged consultants to offer programs like Pathways to Success, as they see the potential return on their investment. Participants did note positive changes in their work, including positive feedback from their manager or others. A potential secondary effect of the workshops may be employee engage-ment, or a tendency to "take the ownership" on the job. From a qualitative perspective, the value of workshop participation for these female profes-sionals was evident.

Descriptive data from SMO evaluation feedback forms evidenced positive perceptions of the SMO participants' satisfaction with the quality of the workshops. Yet the design and use of a different sample prevented the ability to formally triangulate these results with the qualitative findings. An interesting area to explore in future research would be participants' perceived degree of efficacy to affect changes on the job after workshop participation.

CONCLUSION

This exploratory study provides an initial look at professional women in India interacting with an innovative career support intervention. As evidenced by the lack of literature evaluating female talent career support services, especially in emerging markets such as India, this study is rare in explorations of career support workshop responses.

The Pathways to Success workshops, covering a broad array of cognitive, affective, and social interventions to increase women's assertiveness, career planning, branding, use of mentoring, and networking, and other career skills are an important, emerging resource. Designed by women for women professionals, they serve women attempting or expected to rise up through the ranks in or toward senior position, in a country in the midst of a sociocultural and economic revolution.

It is important to note several limitations. First, Pathways to Success modules were not individually evaluated; participants attended one or more modules, and the two interview samples consisted of women who had attended different or overlapping programs. The data, sampling, data collection, and transcribing were conducted by the consultants, drawing upon their program evaluation processes, using industry standard training evaluation forms. The use of in-depth interviews tends to exceed normal business service evaluation. Yet the methodology allows no conclusions on outcomes and only provides a glimpse into workshop participants' responses. Further research is needed to determine the impact of the interventions on women's careers.

The fact that multinational businesses operating in India are motivated to engage consultants to invest in the career development of their female talent is a significant indicator of a positive horizon for professional women. Yet the study also points to the need for recognition of the struggles that women face on a daily basis, and the need to continue expanding options for organizational flexibility and work-life balance resources.

As women enter the workforce in increasing numbers in India, the need to sustain their employment and build their careers, while ensuring their health and well-being, is paramount. If accomplished, a larger social goal will be addressed, as women's employment is associated with gains in maternal and child health, and greater freedoms for women overall (Malhotra, Malhotra, Østbye, & Subramanian, 2012). This speaks to a broader philanthropic social, national, and perhaps global motivation for providing career support services in India.

REFERENCES

Appelbaum, S. H., Asham, N., & Argheyd, K. (2011). Is the glass ceiling cracked in information technology? A qualitative analysis: part 1. *Industrial and Commercial Training, 43*(6), 354–361. doi:10.1108/00197851111160487

Babu, S. S., & Raj, K. B. (2013). Impact of childcare assistance (a work-life balance practice) on employee retention in Indian IT sector. *Global Journal of Management and Business Research, 13*(6). Retrieved from http://www.journalofbusiness.org/index.php/GJMBR/article/view/1039

Baral, R., & Bhargava, S. (2010). Work-family enrichment as a mediator between organizational interventions for work-life balance and job outcomes. *Journal of Managerial Psychology, 25*(3), 274–300. doi:10.1108/02683941011023749.

Bekhouch, Y., Hausmann, R., Tyson, L. D., & Zahidi, S. (2013). *The global gender gap report 2013.* Geneva, Switzerland: World Economic Forum 2013.

Boyar, S. L., & Mosley, D. C. (2007). The relationship between core self-evaluations and work and family satisfaction: The mediating role of work-family conflict and facilitation. *Journal of Vocational Behavior, 71*(2), 265–281.

Bozionelos, N., Bozionelos, G., Kostopoulos, K., & Polychroniou, P. (2011). How providing mentoring relates to career success and organizational commitment: a study in the general managerial population. *Career Development International, 16*(5), 446–468. doi:10.1108/13620431111167760.

Bradwick, J. (1980). The seasons of a woman's life. In D. G. McGuigan (Ed.), *Women's lives: New theory, research and policy.* Ann Arbor, MI: The University of Michigan Press.

Bronfenbrenner, U. (1986). Ecology of the family as a context for human development: Research perspectives. *Developmental Psychology, 22*(6), 723.

Buddhapriya, S. (2009). Work-family challenges and their impact on career decisions: A study of Indian women professionals. *Vikalpa: The Journal for Decision Makers, 34*(1), 31–45.

Budhwar, P. S., Saini, D. S., & Bhatnagar, J. (2005). Women in management in the new economic environment: The case of India. *Asia Pacific Business Review, 11*(2), 179–193. doi:10.1080/1360238042000291199/

Claramma, T. K. (2007). *Work-life balance: A sociological study of women professionals in Kerala* (Unpublished doctoral dissertation).

Delina, G., & Raya, R. P. (2013). A study on work-life balance in working women. *International Journal of Commerce, Business and Management, 2*(5), 274–282.

Desai, M., Majumdar, B., Chakraborty, T., & Ghosh, K. (2011). The second shift: working women in India. *Gender in Management: An International Journal, 26*(6), 432–450. doi:10.1108/17542411111164920.

Dworkin, T. M., Maurer, V., & Schipani, C. A. (2012). Career mentoring for women: New horizons/Expanded methods. *Business Horizons, 55*(4), 363–372. doi:10.1016/j.bushor.2012.03.001.

Ely, R. J., Ibarra, H., & Kolb, D. M. (2011). Taking gender into account: theory and design for women's leadership development programs. *Academy of Management Learning & Education, 10*(3), 474–493.

Gandhi, M. (2013). Glass ceiling for Indian women: Problems and remedies. *Intercontinental Journal of Human Resource Research Review, 1*(6), 12–16.

Gupta, A., Koshal, M., & Koshal, R. K. (1998). Women managers in India: Challenges and opportunities. *Equal Opportunities International, 17*(8), 14–26. doi: 10.1108/02610159810785593

Haynes, R. K., & Ghosh, R. (2012). Towards mentoring the Indian organizational woman: Propositions, considerations, and first steps. *Journal of World Business, 47*(2), 186–193. doi:10.1016/j.jwb.2011.04.005.

Hewlett, S. A., Rashid, R., Leader-Chivee, L., & Fredman, C. (2010). *The battle for female talent in India.* Center for Work-Life Policy. Retrieved from http://asiasociety.org/policy/social-issues/women-and-gender/battle-female-talent-india

Hossen, M. A. (2005). Empowerment-based social work. *The Indian Journal of Social Work, 66*(2), 196–210.

International Institute for Population Sciences and Macro International. (2007). *National Family Health Survey (NFHS-3), 2005–06: India.* Mumbai, India: International Institute for Population Sciences. Retrieved from http://hetv.org/india/nfhs/

Jawahar, I. M., & Hemmasi, P. (2006). Perceived organizational support for women's advancement and turnover intentions: The mediating role of job and employer satisfaction. *Women in Management Review, 21*(8), 643–661. doi:10.1108/09649420610712036

Krishna, C. G. (2013). Career re-launch for mid-life women. *Reflections Journal of Management, 2*(1), 15–21.

Lahoti, R. (2013). Economic growth and female labour force participation in India (Working Paper No. 414). Indian Institute of Management Bangalore. Retrieved from http://www.iimb.ernet.in/research/working-papers/economic-growth-and-female-labour-force-participation-india

Luke, N., & Munshi, K. (2011). Women as agents of change: Female income and mobility in India. *Journal of Development Economics, 94*(1), 1–17. doi:10.1016/j.jdeveco.2010.01.002.

Malhotra, C., Malhotra, R., Østbye, T., & Subramanian, S. V. (2012). Maternal autonomy and child health care utilization in India: results from the National Family Health Survey. *Asia-Pacific Journal of Public Health, 26*(4), 401–413. doi:10.1177/1010539511420418

Naqvi, F. (2011). Perspectives of Indian women managers in the public sector. *Indian Journal of Gender Studies, 18*(3), 279–309. doi:10.1177/097152151101800301/

Nath, D. (2000). Gently shattering the glass ceiling: Experiences of Indian women managers. *Women in Management Review, 15*(1), 44–52. doi:10.1108/09649420010310191

The Nielsen Company. (2011). *Nielsen Women of Tomorrow Study.* Retrieved from http://www.nielsen.com/us/en/press-room/2011/women-of-tomorrow.html

Patel, R., & Parmentier, M. J. C. (2005). The persistence of traditional gender roles in the information technology sector: A study of female engineers in India. *Information Technologies and International Development, 2*(3), 29–46. doi:10.1162/1544752054782457.

Society for Human Resource Management. (2009). *Perspectives on women in management in India.* Retrieved from http://www.shrm.org/research/articles/articles/documents/09-0677_india_women_ldrshp_fnl.pdf

Srinivasan, V., Murty, L. S., & Nakra, M. (2013). Career persistence of women software professionals in India. *Gender in Management: An International Journal, 28*(4), 210–227. doi:10.1108/GM-01-2013-0011.

Tan, F. Y., & Yahya, K. K. (2013). Career planning and career strategy: A study of Malaysian insurance agents. *International Proceedings of Economics Development & Research, 55*, 17–22. doi:10.7763/IPEDR.2012.V55. 4.

Tarr-Whelan, L. (2009). *Women lead the way: Your guide to stepping up to leadership and changing the world.* San Francisco, CA: Berrett-Koehler Publishers.

Wayne, J. H., Randel, A. E., & Stevens, J. (2006). The role of identity and work–family support in work–family enrichment and its work-related consequences. *Journal of Vocational Behavior, 69*(3), 445–461.

Williams, J. C. (2004). Hitting the maternal wall. *Academe, 90*(6), 16–20.

Valk, R., & Srinivasan, V. (2011). Work–family balance of Indian women software professionals: A qualitative study. *IIMB Management Review, 23*(1), 39–50. doi:10.1016/j.iimb.2010.10.010.

A Substance Abuse Intervention Program at a Large Russian Manufacturing Worksite

KENNETH BURGESS, MEd

Corporate Health Russia, Brenham, Texas

RICHARD LENNOX, PhD, and DAVID A. SHARAR, PhD

Chestnut Global Partners, Bloomington, Illinois

ALEXANDER SHTOULMAN, MD

Corporate Health Russia, Moscow, Russia

Motivating alcohol abusers to enter treatment, comply with recommendations, and make significant changes in their behavior is no easy task. In the West, professionals learned the importance of motivation early on, and they learned it first from those recovering in Alcoholics Anonymous. Early occupational alcoholism programs used job performance and disciplinary steps to motivate problem drinkers to take action. The threat of job loss proved significant in breaking through denial and in motivating clients to begin a recovery process. This approach was incorporated into the Employee Assistance Program (EAP) and EAP professionals have used job performance and disciplinary steps to motivate those with many types of personal issues. In the Russian Federation, no such history exists. This workplace-based alcohol intervention program is a first for Russia, and it uses the work performance approach successfully deployed in the West for many decades.

Color versions of one or more of the figures in the article can be found online at www.tandfonline.com/wjwb.

INTRODUCTION

There is no question as to the extent that alcohol abuse negatively affects the quantity and quality of human life. Studies have also linked alcohol consumption to all types of unintentional injuries (Hingson & Howland, 1993; Ridolfo & Stevenson, 2001). Although questions remain pertaining to the actual link between alcohol use and abuse on and off the job, and injuries and fatalities at the workplace, research continues to show that the involvement of alcohol in unintentional injury is high (Gmel & Rehm, 2003). From the literature we find that alcohol is frequently found in the blood (blood alcohol content) of those being treated for injury, and cumulative findings from many studies position the drug as having at least some causal role.

Alcohol use disorders (AUDs) have been significantly underestimated and undertreated by health professionals in the Russian Federation (Gmel & Rehm, 2003; Nemtsov, 2000; Korolenko, Minevich, & Segal, 1994; Pridemore, 2002). From the World Health Organization (WHO; 2011) we learn that AUDs rank seventh among the leading causes of premature death and disability worldwide. The countries with the highest alcohol usage are clustered in Eastern Europe, particularly Russia and among the countries of the former Soviet Union (WHO, 2014). Moldova, for example, ranks first in the world (WHO, 2014). In addition, alcohol dependence has been established to rank as number 12 of the leading 20 causes of death worldwide (Mathers, Boerma, & Ma Fat, 2009; Rehm, Gmel, Sempos, & Trevisan, 2003). Important to this study, cultural differences do appear to play a role in drinking, particularly with regard to how much one drinks, when one drinks, and where one drinks (WHO, 2007).

According to the Russian government, alcohol consumption is more than double the critical level set by the WHO at 8 liters of ethanol per-individual annually (Ria Novasti, 2009). And Russia has long exceeded this level of consumption. On September 11, 2009, then-President Dmitry Medvedev ordered his government to prepare draft laws to counter alcohol abuse.

The heavy use of alcohol certainly impairs job performance and safety and results in expensive medical, social, and related personal problems affecting employee lives, productivity, and families. Productivity losses in Russia have not been officially quantified, but elsewhere, such losses have been estimated at billions of euros/dollars annually. Drug use is also on the rise in Russia, adding to workplace concerns.

The alcohol intervention program that was developed at this Russian industrial site deals directly with these issues using methodologies proven effective at other world locations. Western companies recognized the importance of addressing alcohol abuse early on, and today we learn from the Society for Human Resource Management (2008) that almost 90% of large organizations in the United States (those with more than 500 employees) have some type of workplace intervention service in place. This was a strong selling point for management at this Russian company who were concerned about the problem at their worksites, and concerned too, about their government's announcements as to the extent of the problem in Russia.

Alcohol Interventions in a Resource-Limited Setting

The implementation of an alcohol intervention service in a resource-limited region presents problems. The models in place elsewhere reflect the work of alcoholism specialists where there have traditionally been a great deal of treatment resources available. Treatment services are scarce in Russia, particularly outside of the large metropolitan areas of St. Petersburg and Moscow. In the region where this program operates, services were almost nonexistent. You will see how this program addressed these concerns by putting a great deal of time and effort into training local medical professionals, company management, and others from the community.

The Advantage of the Workplace Setting

In the West, beginning first in the United States as early as 1940, workplaces proved to be ideal locations from which to provide alcohol intervention. Workers spend a great deal of their time "on the job" and employers have well-developed means at their disposal to deal with problem drinkers (Roman & Bloom, 2002; Roman & Trice, 1972).

The goal of the industrial alcoholism program is to use corrective action (discipline) to confront an employee and to facilitate a corrective action intervention. The program at this location uses this approach, maintaining the employee's job while the employee receives necessary treatment, and corrective action continues should the employee fail to adhere to recommendations: up to and including termination. Work plays a very important role in one's life. Because the adults' role in a family is to maintain an income, employers have a substantial amount of leverage. And, one's overall status and prestige in society, particularly for men, is largely based on one's employment (Gannett, 2013). We began our work for this company with these concepts in mind and implemented the company's Alcohol Program based on an approach that made earlier programming in the West successful. No such effort has ever been implemented in the Russian Federation, and this employer is receiving country-wide recognition for the results achieved.

HOW THE PROGRAM WORKS

The Program Professional

At this industrial worksite, there is a full-time employee who serves as the program interventionist. A local female social worker with limited prior experience in alcoholism treatment, the company's interventionist was trained by the professional staff at Corporate Health (CH). The CH director in Moscow, a physician, has substantial knowledge and experience in the addictions field, having also completed training in this area in the United States. A Russian, he also fully understood the challenges the company faced in putting this service in place. The program interventionist was trained at the CH offices in Moscow, and during the first year of operation she received regular, ongoing telephonic clinical supervision from the CH staff. She also received input and guidance from the partner organizations in the United States.

The interventionist provides a diagnostic, referral and follow-up service to those referred by supervisors, managers, Human Resources (HR) and medical representatives. All such referrals are based on work performance, safety violations, and/or health concerns. Employees are guided to the service by their immediate supervisor (or an HR or medical official). These referrals are firm, but the employee does have the right to reject help. Should work problems continue, a stronger referral is made with the employee expected to follow the interventionist's recommendation(s). In the event that an initial violation is severe, that is, a major violation, the employee is expected to present himself or herself to the interventionist in lieu of being terminated. And, those who are terminated are referred back to the program as part of the termination process. Such employees are told that "they may have an opportunity to return to work, but only after they complete the program successfully."

There are generally four types of referrals made to the program:

1. Self-referral: Employees seek help from the interventionist on their own. The identity of the employee is kept highly confidential and while expected to complete the program offered, adherence is voluntary.
2. "Soft" or "recommended" referral: Employees with less severe performance problems are asked by their supervisor to contact the program and work with the interventionist. The referring supervisor is kept informed (through a signed release of information) as to the employee's compliance.
3. Formal referral: The employee is referred in lieu of being terminated with successful completion of the services expected. Failure to complete services results in termination.
4. Formal referral after termination: Employees who are terminated are referred back to the program and expected to complete services to be eligible for rehire.

The results of such referrals appear in the research findings.

The Intervention Team

We involved all medical professionals (contractors) who worked for the company in a 4-day team-building training effort. A number of community-based medical professionals also participated. This training was directed by the CH program director (a physician) and included input from a U.S. physician consultant, a psychiatrist highly skilled in addiction, who participated using an Internet connection:

- Physicians and nurses reviewed internationally recognized criteria for the diagnosis of alcohol and other substance dependency with the program director and U.S. consultant.
- Methods of drug/alcohol detection were presented and discussed.
- Medical intervention points were presented and discussed.
- The interventionist was introduced and her role clearly defined.

A small local treatment group (of five psychologists) received a similar training. The medical training was conducted at the local hospital; the other sessions were held at the city's municipal offices. This effort was fully supported by the town mayor and her government team.

To ensure local support, we held one-hour introductory presentations at City Hall and invited the media, law enforcement, the clergy, school officials, and others from the community to attend. We also presented the program to the company's union representatives, and they, in turn, hosted six "open" sessions with union membership at the union hall. And, we attended five "open" Alcoholics Anonymous (AA) meetings to ask for understanding and assistance from those who best understood the problem. Although still formative, we found AA to be growing in this region of Russia, and we also found strong support for this effort from the recovering community.

The Plant Program Committee

An in-plant Program Committee was initiated with management and the union. This Committee has 12 members and represents a cross-section of the various departments/groups found at the plant.

The Committee was initiated with high-level representatives from management, HR, social services, safety, medical, and the union as members. This group developed the program policies and procedures for the plant. After the completion of their work, this high-level representative appointed an individual from their division to serve on the Committee. This Committee met monthly for the first 6 months of operation but now holds its meetings quarterly. (Although, they do meet according to need, and special meetings are often called to address any emergent issue.) The clearly defined role of those serving on the Committee is to provide program support, recommendations, and to address any concerns that may arise. They do not provide any clinical input or direction.

Program Policies/Procedures

HR policies and procedures were revised to support this intervention effort. The Committee reviewed policy/procedural statements from Western organizations and revised accordingly. Corporate Health (and its U.S. organizations) provided consultation during this effort. Ongoing program operational procedures (including a program manual) were developed and the Initial Program Committee was established. This "initial" Program Committee developed position descriptions and guidelines for the follow up Committee. The Intervention Program became operational on May 1, 2011, after the completion of all of the (above) action steps.

Evaluation of the Program

Our study compared 66 workers referred to the Intervention Program who were identified as having drinking problems with 338 workers from the general population of a similar company (control group). Both received a questionnaire containing measures of alcohol use, absenteeism, presenteeism, work engagement, life satisfaction, and workplace distress. This comparison formed a 2 × 2 mixed factorial research design. The treatment condition (experimental vs. control) was a between-groups factor and time (pretreatment vs. follow-up) was a within-subject factor. The treatment hypothesis was that the treatment and control conditions would differ at baseline reflecting the fact that the treatment group had identified alcohol problems, with a control group representing the general population. Program effectiveness would presumably remove the difference between these groups at follow-up. These hypotheses were tested using an analysis of variance. Support for the hypotheses would be expected to produce a statistically significant interaction between the treatment group and time factors.

Research Design

This study used a quasi-experimental design with non-equivalent groups. Two groups were compared: the treatment group receiving the intervention/ program at one company site and a control group from another similar company work location, with a work population similar in age, gender, and other important demographics.

Using a pretest/posttest design, we tracked the changes in the outcome measures via a repeated measures component. With this design, the participants also served as their own controls. The design used a covariate analysis to remove preexisting differences in outcome measures caused simply by differences in comparison between the groups.

Measures

The full Global Appraisal of Individual Needs (GAIN) is a standardized and scientifically validated biopsychosocial tool that integrates clinical and research assessment for people presenting to behavioral health treatment (Dennis, Titus, White, Unsicker, & Hodgkins, 2003). It asks about symptoms from the *Diagnostic and Statistical Manual of Mental Disorders, Fourth Edition* (*DSM-IV-TR; with changed code*) that can be used to generate dimensional symptom count measures or categorical diagnostic impressions of specific disorder in the four main dimensions of interest (i.e., internalizing, externalizing, substance, and crime/violence). Although well received (it is currently used by more than 750 agencies across the United States, Canada, and Mexico), it typically takes 2 to 3 months of training and feedback to get a staff person certified on GAIN administration and then takes 90 to 120 minutes per patient/staff person to actually administer. This takes too much time for use as a screener in settings like the workplace or Internet-based health risk assessments where it may only be one of several components and there is limited time or limited staff resources. Thus, there was a need to develop a GAIN-Short Screener (GAIN-SS) that could be (a) easily trained, (b) used in 5 minutes or fewer to identify people who have a disorder and rule out people who do not, and c) provide guidance for referral to further assessment and treatment. Consistent with the full GAIN, the GAIN-SS (Dennis, Chan, & Funk, 2006; Dennis, Feeney, & Titus, 2006). is designed to (a) be valid for adolescent and adult populations, (b) provide measures of severity overall and the four main dimensions of emotional/behavioral problems (internalizing, externalizing, substance, crime/violence), and (c) triage these dimensions to provide guides to support clinical decision making about detailed diagnosis and treatment needs. In this particular study, the crime/violence scale of the GAIN-SS was eliminated at the request of the sponsoring multinational employers who permitted the use of the other GAIN-SS scales among its expatriate or U.S. domestic workforce.

The 3- to 5-minute GAIN-SS, the instrument used in this study, was designed to serve as a screener in general populations to quickly and accurately identify clients whom the full 1.5- to 2-hour full GAIN would identify as having one or more behavioral health disorders (e.g., internalizing or externalizing psychiatric disorders, substance use disorders, or crime/violence problems), which would suggest the need for a referral to a mental health professional. It also rules out those who would not be identified as having behavioral health disorders. The GAIN-SS is designed for self-or staff administration with paper and pen, on a computer, or on the web.

GAIN-SS responses are given in terms of the recency of the problem described in the questions: 3 (*past month*), 2 (*2 to 12 months ago*), 1 (*1 + years ago*), 0 (*never*). The number of past-month symptoms (number of 3's) is used as a measure of change; the number of past-year symptoms (number of 3's or 2's) is used to identify who is likely to have a current diagnosis; and the number of lifetime symptoms (number of 3's, 2's, or 1's) is used as a covariate measure of lifetime severity. The recency measures can also be combined to create course specifics (e.g., early remission means having a lifetime problem but not in the past month; sustained remission means having a lifetime problem but not in the past year).

Dennis et al. (2006) found that for adolescents and adults the 20-item total disorder screener and its 45-item subscreeners (internalizing disorders, externalizing disorders, substance disorders, and crime/violence) have good internal consistency (alpha of .96 on the total screener), were highly correlated ($r = .84$ to .94) with the 123-item scales in the full GAIN, had excellent sensitivity (90% or more) for identifying people with a disorder, and excellent specificity (92% or more) for correctly ruling out people who did not have a disorder.

A confirmatory factor analysis of the structure of the GAIN-SS showed that it is also consistent with the full GAIN after allowing adolescent and adult path coefficients to vary and cross-loading paths between conduct disorder items with crime/violence items. The confirmatory factor analysis was slightly less accurate than the full-scale version in terms of the Confirmatory Fit Index (CFI; .87 for the GAIN-SS vs. .92 for the full GAIN, whereas the CFI approaches 1 the model fits the data better), and slightly more precise in terms of the root mean square error of approximation (RMSEA; .05 for GAIN-SS vs. .06 for the full GAIN, whereas the RMSEA goes down there is less unexplained variance). This suggests that each of the subscreeners has good discriminate validity and that the total structure is consistent with the model used with the full GAIN.

It is generally believed that the strongest evaluation design for a program-level intervention involves a random assignment of participants to a treatment condition and an isolated no-treatment or alternative control condition with an active manipulation of the independent variable. Such an approach is generally regarded as a "true experiment" in that it assures that posttreatment change is unequivocally linked to the treatment program and not extraneous factors, and as such, benefits from strong internal validity. Unfortunately, random assignment to isolated treatment and control condition is difficult to achieve in real-world setting without creating a contrived situation that is low in external validity. For example, medical studies that test the efficacy of the treatment in laboratory settings often fail to appreciate the complications of the operational environment in which the programs exist and thus fail in field implementation. Regarding workplace-based alcohol interventions, failure to consider the complications of workplace implementation is likely to create a sterile program that does not adhere to the real world. Because it is not feasible to randomly assign workers to a treatment and control condition, we employed a quasi-experimental design that tracked the changes in outcome(s), tracking those who used the service against those who did not.

The evaluation design was a 2×2 within-subjects design, using an experimental group that received the intervention (and were questioned before services began), then questioned again 90 days after their intervention. The control group (workers from another similar company site) did not receive an intervention and did not receive program services. The controls were questioned at the beginning of the study and were then (follow up) questioned approximately 120 days after their initial questioning. This 30-day differential allowed for the passage of time for the experimental group and created roughly an equal pre-treatment posttreatment lag.

A Russian language version of the short screener of the GAIN-SS along with the Substance Problem Index and the Substance Frequency Scale from the GAIN served as the primary behavioral health outcome measures for this study and tested the primary hypotheses regarding the effectiveness of the program in reducing alcohol use. A newly translated version of the Workplace Outcome Suite (WOS), which included self-report measures of absenteeism, presenteeism, work engagement, life satisfaction, and workplace distress was used to test secondary outcomes related to improvements in workplace functioning and quality of life measures.

The WOS provides secondary outcome measures of absenteeism, presenteeism, work engagement, life satisfaction, and workplace distress with which to measures secondary outcomes (Lennox, Sharar, Schmitz, & Goehner, 2010). This 5-item measure is a psychometrically derived version of a longer scale questionnaire (25 items) aimed at assessing quality of life issues surrounding productivity in the workplace and at home.

Another secondary measure used was the World Health Organization's 10-item Alcohol Use Disorders Identification Test (AUDIT) which helped to provide us with ancillary measures of alcohol problems and alcohol dependence (Saunders, Aasland, Babor, de la Fuente, & Grant, 1993).

Participants

Participants were 66 workers from a single worksite who received the intervention (the experimental group), and another 330 workers from a similar site who served as the treatment control group.

Procedures

Upon referral to the program, treatment participants received an intake interview during which the baseline variables were collected. The exact treatment services that individual workers received was determined by the treatment professional at the program. To standardize the effects of the study, treatment subjects were reassessed (posttreatment follow-up) 90 days after their entry into the program, regardless of the actual services they received. Control participants at the control site were randomly recruited and did not receive any services from the program. The control participants were followed up with the questionnaire at approximately 120 days.

Statistical Analysis

The main hypotheses was tested using an analysis of covariance (ANCOVA) of the average scores on outcome measures at the 90-day follow-up for the treatment group; 120 days for the controls. Baseline alcohol use measures from the Social Functioning Scale were used to remove the effect of pretreatment differences between the treatment group/controls regarding their (initial) alcohol intake. Type III sums of squares were used to implement the statistical controls for any preexisting differences. Table 1 presents the descriptive statistics for the items in all questionnaires used in this study.

In this quasi-experimental study we compare a general control groups that is expected to have the normal amount of alcohol problems with an experimental groups specifically selected to be in need of an alcohol intervention. The main test of the effectiveness of the intervention is necessarily an overall lack of alcohol use and/or problem, but rather a return to a state that is similar to a general population. Because the treatment group was selected for its alcohol problems, we expect it to show more alcohol use and workplace dysfunction than the more heterogeneous control group. There should be some differences between the two groups at intake, but we expect these differences to statistically disappear to at least be substantially less at the follow-up assessment.

Absenteeism and self-reported alcohol use in the past 30 days among the 66 treatment participants did not produce enough variance to allow statistical tests of the hypotheses. None of the 66 participants reported any alcohol uses during that time, and on the surface this finding supports the efficacy of the program. However, the fact that none of the participants reported any use needs to be carefully considered. It is possible that participants were unwilling to admit to any alcohol use. It is also possible that the threat of being fired for drinking was so potent as to provide sufficient motivation to remain abstinent. Only 2 of the 66 participants reported any absenteeism during the 90-day follow-up period. Here again, such a uniform lack of absenteeism is extremely rare in social research. Taken together, the two variables raise some question about the veracity of the report, but they cannot by themselves vitiate the results. A post hoc interview of the 66 treatment participants may be useful in providing insight into the validity of the self-reported measures of alcohol use and absenteeism. It may also be useful to conduct informal interviews of the supervisors of a small subset of the treatment participants. It is worth noting that the interventionist collecting the reports did not get the impression that the participants were providing false reports of either of these variables.

TABLE 1 Descriptive Statistics of the Pretreatment Questionnaire (Treatment Group, $n = 66$)

	% Yes	% No
GAIN Short Screener (Substance Use Disorder Screener)		
1. You used alcohol or other drugs weekly or more often?	63.6	36.4
2. You spent a lot of time either getting alcohol or other drugs, using alcohol or other drugs, or feeling the effects of alcohol or other drugs?	9.1	90.9
3. You kept using alcohol or other drugs even though it was causing social problems, leading to fights, or getting you into trouble with other people?	19.7	19.7
4. Your use of alcohol or other drugs caused you to give up, reduce or have problems at important activities at work, school, home, or social events?	33.3	66.7
5. You had withdrawal problems from alcohol or other drugs like shaky hands, throwing up, having trouble sitting still or sleeping, or that you used any alcohol or other drugs to stop being sick or avoid withdrawal problems?	39.4	60.6

	% 0	% 4
Alcohol Use Disorders Identification Test		
1. How many times do you have a drink containing alcohol?	3.0	9.1
2. How many drinks containing alcohol do you have on a typical day when you are drinking?	6.1	13.6
3. How often do you have six or more drinks on one occasion?	9.1	0.0
4. How often during the last year have you found that you were not able to stop drinking once you had started?	40.9	1.5
5. How often during the last year have you failed to do what was normally expected of you because of drinking?	47.0	3.0
6. How often during the last year have you needed a first drink in the morning to get yourself going after a heavy drinking session?	47.0	0.0
7. How often during the last year have you had a feeling of guilt or remorse after drinking?	19.7	6.1
8. How often during the last year have you been unable to remember what happened the night before because of your drinking?	45.5	0.0
9. Have you or someone else been injured because of your drinking?	75.8	9.1
10. Has a relative, friend, doctor, or other health care worker been concerned about your drinking or suggested you cut down?	19.7	72.7

	M	SD
Workplace Outcome Suite (5-Item Version)		
1. For the period of the past thirty (30) days, please total the number of hours your drinking caused you to miss work including complete 8-hour days and partial days when you came in late or left early.	6.52	12.15
2. My personal problems keep me from concentrating on my work.	2.86	1.51
3. I am often eager to get to the work site to start the day.	2.79	1.18
4. So far, my life seems to be going very well.	2.73	1.26
5. I dread going into work.	2.85	1.63

Note. GAIN = Global Appraisal of Individual Needs.

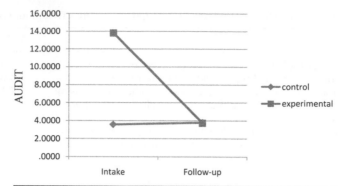

	Condition	Intake	Follow-up
	Control	3.5905	3.7959
Mean	Experimental	13.7879	3.7576
	Total	5.2605	3.7896
	0 Control	337	338
N	1 Experimental	66	66
	Total	403	404
	0 Control	4.36964	4.28887
SD	1 Experimental	6.65759	2.63153
	Total	6.11573	4.06190

FIGURE 1 Descriptive statistics of Alcohol Use Disorders Identification Test (AUDIT) scores for treatment and control groups at intake and follow-up.

Figure 1 presents the results of the tests of the treatment hypotheses for the AUDIT alcohol outcomes measures. As shown in the figures there are substantial differences between the 66 participants in the treatment group (experimental) and the 337 in the control group at the beginning of the study on the AUDIT measures. These differences reflect the fact that the treatment group was selected for their apparent misuse of alcohol and its adverse impact on job performance. However, as shown in Figure 1 and the table these differences essentially disappear after treatment, indicating that the intervention brought the AUDIT scores to a level consistent with the general working population.

The test of the statistical interaction between condition and time was statistically significant ($F = 145.630$ (1, 803), $p < .000$) indicating that the slope of the lines presented in the graph are different from one another and specifically that steep declining slope for the treatment group suggesting a pronounced reduction on the AUDIT scores from intake to follow-up is very different from the relatively flat line for the control group. The treatment group decreased from intake to follow-up to the point where they were statistically equivalent to the control group, and thus the treatment group was essentially returned to the normal state of the general population. The results of the core analysis provide the strongest support for the alcohol program's ability to ameliorate the drinking problem in this group.

We used an ANCOVA implemented with Type III sums of squares to statistically control for the possibility that the treatment and control groups contained pretreatment differences that would confound the outcome differences. A Type II sums of squares was used to partial out any variance in the outcome variables attributed to pretreatment differences between treatment and control groups.

Figure 2 presents the intake and follow-up patterns for the presenteeism scale with high scores indicating that one's alcoholism has an adverse effect on work. Lowers score therefore indicate better functioning. Unlike the

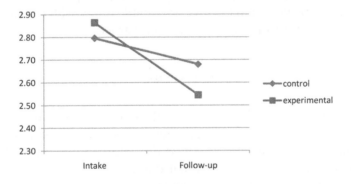

	Condition	Intake	Follow-up
	Control	3.5905	3.7959
Mean	Experimental	13.7879	3.7576
	Total	5.2605	3.7896
	0 Control	337	338
N	1 Experimental	66	66
	Total	403	404
	0 Control	4.36964	4.28887
SD	1 Experimental	6.65759	2.63153
	Total	6.11573	4.06190

FIGURE 2 Descriptive statistics of presenteeism scores for treatment and control groups at intake and follow-up.

AUDIT the presenteeism score at intake for the two groups is quite small. However, the score diverge at follow-up, to the point where the treatment shows the better functioning. On the surface, this pattern of means also shows support the for treatment hypotheses in showing that the treatment group improved at a better rate than the control did, finally achieving the lowest score for all comparison. That is, though the treatment group initially showed the highest amount of adverse effect on the job, by the end of the follow-up it was the lowest.

The background statistics, however, show that these differences are not statistically different, and thus do not provide strong support for the treatment hypotheses ($F = .463$ (1, 804), $p = .497$). However, because of the small sample, this test did not provide adequate statistical power for the presenteeism effect. The observed power statistic in the appendix gauges the statistical power of the test on a scale of 0 to 1.00, with 0 being a *total lack of power* and 1.00 being *very high statistical power*. The observed power of .104 suggests that the sample was just not large enough to provide a sensitive test of the presenteeism effect, and thus we are unable to say with certainty whether the treatment can affect presenteeism as a construct.

SUMMARY

This study evaluated the efficacy of workplace alcohol interventions by comparing the alcohol use and workplace outcomes of 66 workers identified as having drinking problems who received the intervention, with 338 workers from the general population of a similar company (the control group). Both groups received a questionnaire containing measures of alcohol use, absenteeism, presenteeism, work engagement, life satisfaction, and workplace distress. This comparison formed a 2×2 mixed factorial research design. The treatment condition (experimental vs. control) was a between-groups factor and time (pretreatment versus follow-up) was a within-subject factor. The treatment hypothesis was that the treatment and control conditions would differ at baseline reflecting the fact that the treatment group had identified alcohol problems, with the control group representing the general population. Program effectiveness would presumably remove the difference between these groups at follow-up. The hypotheses were tested using an analysis of variance. Support for the hypotheses would be expected to produce a statistically significant interaction between the treatment group and time factors.

Statistically significant interaction for the AUDIT scores and life satisfaction clearly supported the effectiveness of the program by showing that large differences between the experimental and control groups at baseline essentially disappeared at follow-up. The results of the follow-up survey for the experimental group suggested that there was no self-reported drinking and little absenteeism 30 days after intervention. The low variance in these measures precluded formal statistical analysis. The pattern seen favored the effectiveness of the intervention. Workplace outcomes measures for work engagement and workplace distress showed the same pattern but did not reach traditional levels of statistical significance. The results of the presentee-ism scale did not support the hypothesis.

The results of the primary outcome measures provided strong support for this intervention. Large differences on the AUDIT between the high scores for the experimental group and the low scores for the general population (control group) essentially disappeared at follow-up. The consistent pattern for mean-differences in all but the presenteeism scale suggests that the sample size was not large to permit a sensitive testing of the hypotheses and that if additional participants had been provided there would have been stronger evidence in support of the intervention. However, it is impressive to note that positive evidence emerged even with this small sampling. The results of our work suggests that continuing this research using larger samples (300 or more individuals within each group) could provide an extremely robust statement of the effectiveness of the workplace alcohol program in Russia.

REFERENCES

Dennis, M. L., Chan, Y.-F., & Funk, R. R. (2006). Development and validation of the GAIN Short Screener (GSS) for internalizing, externalizing and substance use disorders and crime/violence problems among adolescents and adults. *American Journal on Addictions, 15,* 80–91. doi: 10.1080/10550490601006055

Dennis, M. L., Feeney, T., & Titus, J. C. (2006). *Global Appraisal of Individual Needs Short Screener (GAIN-SS): Administration and scoring manual version 3.* Normal, IL: Chestnut Health Systems. Retrieved from http://www.gaincc.org/_data/files/Instruments%20and%20Reports/Instruments%20Manuals/GAIN-SS_Manual_3_0.pdf

Dennis, M. L., Titus, J. C., White, M., Unsicker, J., & Hodgkins, D. (2003). *Global Appraisal of Individual Needs (GAIN): Administration guide for the GAIN and related measures.* Bloomington, IL: Chestnut Health Systems. Retrieved from http://www.gaincc.org/_data/files/Instruments%20and%20Reports/Instruments%20Manuals/GAIN-I%20manual_combined_0512.pdf

Gannett, A. K. (2013, August 31). At work: Job, self-esteem tied tightly together. *USA Today.* Retrieved from http://www.usatoday.com/story/money/columnist/kay/2013/08/31/at-work-self-esteem-depression/2736083/

Gmel, G., & Rehm, J. (2003). *Harmful alcohol use.* National Institute on Alcohol Abuse and Alcoholism (NIH). Retrieved from http://pubs.niaaa.nih.gov/publications/Arh27-1/52-62.htm

Hingson, R., & Howland, J. (1993). Alcohol and non–traffic unintended injuries. *Addiction, 88*(7), 877–883.

Korolenko, C., Minevich, V., & Segal, B. (1994). The politicization of alcohol in the USSR and its impact on the study and treatment of alcoholism. *International Journal of Addiction, 29,* 1269–1285.

Lennox, R., Sharar, D., Schmitz, E., & Goehner, D. (2010). Development and validation of the Chestnut Workplace Outcome Suite. *Journal of Workplace Behavioral Health, 25,* 107–131.

Mathers, C. D., Boerma, T., & Ma Fat, D. (2009). Global and regional causes of death. *British Medical Bulletin, 92,* 7–32.

Nemtsov, A. V. (2000). Estimates of total alcohol consumption in Russia, 1920–1994. *Drug and Alcohol Dependence, 58,* 133–142.

Pridemore, A. W. (2002). Vodka and violence: Alcohol consumption and homicide rates in Russia. *American Journal of Public Health, 92*(12), 1921–1930.

Rehm, J., Gmel, G., Sempos, C. T., & Trevisan, M. (2003). *Alcohol-related morbidity and mortality.* National Institute on Alcohol Abuse and Alcoholism (NIAAA) – NIH. Retrieved from http://pubs.niaaa.nih.gov/publications/arh27-1/3

Ria Novasti – the Russian Agency of International Information. (2009). *Alcoholic Russia.* October 14th edition. Retrieved at https://larussophobe.wordpress.com/2009/10/11/october-14-2009-contents/

Ridolfo, B., & Stevenson, C. (2001). *DRUG STATISTICS SERIES Number 7: The quantification of drug–caused mortality and morbidity in Australia, 1998.* Canberra, Australia: Australian Institute of Health and Welfare. Retrieved from http://www.aihw.gov.au/WorkArea/DownloadAsset.aspx?id=6442459309

Roman, P., & Bloom, T. (2002). *The workplace and alcohol problem prevention.* National Institute on Alcohol Abuse and Alcoholism (NIAAQA) - NIH. Retrieved from http://pubs.niaaa.nih.gov/publications/arh26-1/49-57.htm

Roman, P. M., & Trice, H. M. (1972). *Spirits and demons at work.* New York State School of Industrial and Labor Relations, Cornell University, B007EPOM2G.

Saunders, J. B., Aasland, O. G., Babor, T. F., de la Fuente, J. R., & Grant, M. (1993). Development of the Alcohol Use Disorders Identification Test (AUDIT): WHO collaborative project on early detection of persons with harmful alcohol consumption II. *Addiction, 88*(6), 791–804.

Society for Human Resource Management. (2008). *2008 employee benefits: How competitive is your organization? Survey report by the Society of Human Resource Management.* Retrieved from http://www.shrm.org/research/surveyfindings/documents/08-0335_benefitssr_final_.pdf

World Health Organization (WHO). (2007). *The world health report 2007 – A safer future: Global public health security in the 21st century.* Retrieved from http://www.who.int/whr/2007/en/

World Health Organization (WHO). (2011). *Management of substance abuse: The global burden.* Retrieved from http://www.who.int/substanceabuse/facts/globalburden/en/index.html

World Health Organization (WHO). (2014). *Global status report on alcohol and health 2014.* WHO Library Cataloguing-in-Publication Data. Retrieved from http://apps.who.int/iris/bitstream/10665/112736/1/9789240692763_eng.pdf

Pricing Models of Employee Assistance Programs: Experiences of Corporate Clients Serviced by a Leading Employee Assistance Program Service Provider in South Africa

NELISWA A. CEKISO, MSW, and
LOURENS S. TERBLANCHE, MSW, PhD

Department of Social Work and Criminology, University of Pretoria, Pretoria, South Africa

Pricing is a challenging area in the Employee Assistance Program (EAP) field. The gap identified between theory and practice is the lack of scientific data on typical pricing model practices. This results in a lack of uniformity, which affects negatively on the professional standards of the Employee Assistance field—specifically in the South African situation. Pricing and contracting processes often result in challenges that must be identified timeously by both the EAP service provider and the corporate client. The researchers thus explored the processes and complexities involved in the pricing practices by investigating the experiences of corporate clients and account managers of a leading EAP service provider. The research findings indicate a number of factors that must be considered in the contracting and pricing processes.

INTRODUCTION

"Clients will not pay for services that cannot be justified and they will not work or contract with vendors who cannot meet their needs" (Peters, 1999, p. 84). The statement illustrates some of the possible factors that motivate certain corporate clients to terminate contracts prematurely. However, it should also be noted that, despite the principle of paying for value, as

TABLE 1 Summary of Themes and Sub Themes on Pricing of EAPs

Number	Theme	Subtheme
1	Complexities experienced by a leading EAP service provider and corporate clients in relation to contracting for EAP services within the EAP field	• Competition • Price • Different pricing models • Contracting • Economy
2	Internal processes in preparation for submission of a bid for a contract	• Company's budget • Size of the company • Utilization • Type of services • Relationship with corporate client • Embedded costs
3	Role players involved in the submission of a bid	• Internal role players • External role players
4	External processes encountered in the submission of a bid	• Procurement policies and procedures
5	Quality of services	

Note. EAP = Employee Assistance Program.

demanded by the corporate client, Employee Assistance Program (EAP) service providers are also confronted by the challenge of pricing.

Pricing seems to be driven by what constitutes the selection and implementation of a model for a service. The challenge becomes more complex in situations where clients are quoted differently for the same service. The situation is aggravated by what Sharar (2004) cited as fierce competition and the oversupply of EAP service providers. This oversupply and the competition among competitors have caused many EAP service providers to submit unrealistically low bids, resulting in failure to conform to quality standards and meeting clients' needs. Sharar and Hertenstein (2006) elaborated further, citing the common dilemma that faces corporate clients during procurement processes. The issue of prices has encouraged employers to make their choice based on how little they have to pay. They thus lose sight of the program's original mission, which is its early identification and consequent ability to intervene in maximizing employee productivity and effectiveness in the workplace.

The problem identified, which motivated the researchers to undertake this study, is the lack of scientific data on typical pricing model practices in the EAP field. This results in a lack of uniformity, which affects negatively the professional standards of the EA field. To bridge the identified gap, the authors explored the complexities and processes involved in the pricing models of the EAP field. The study explored the experiences of corporate clients who had terminated contracts with a leading EAP service provider and participants (account managers) from this leading EAP service provider.

EAP PRICING MODELS

Realizing the mission of EAPs requires EAP practitioners and service providers to design programs that will best serve the needs of corporate clients, while taking into consideration the resources that will be required to deliver to their needs. On the other hand, corporate clients should conduct comprehensive organizational assessment if they want a clear understanding of the organizational needs and should plan accordingly in terms of budget allocation (Standards Committee of Employee Assistance Professionals Association of South Africa [EAPA-SA], 2010). This argument is based on the understanding that pricing models determine the actual price that EAP service providers charge for services offered to corporate clients. As the identification of pricing is a problem in the EAP field, this has encouraged employers to choose according to how little they have to pay. However, in the process, they lose sight of the program's original mission, which is early identification and intervention to maximize employee productivity and effectiveness in the workplace (Lee, 2005). Although the argument raised by the authors seems to point to the shortcomings of corporate clients when contracting with EAP service providers, the question to be explored is that of how the EAP service providers have managed to reach the lowest bids and what informed the pricing models that were applied in the preparation of a submission for a bid.

In the literature review for this study, the authors attempted to explore factors considered for pricing in the EAP field which subsequently impact on the choice of pricing models. Marketing as a phenomenon will also be explored, as pricing and the pricing models used in the EAP field are linked to a company's marketing strategy.

FACTORS AFFECTING PRICING IN THE EAP FIELD

Marketing of EAPS

Marketing EAPs is a vehicle for raising awareness and recognition of EAP as a strategic tool for work organizations. Failure to market the program effectively affects negatively the perception of the program, including its resource allocation. Winegar (2002) identified marketing, particularly the marketing and selling of EAPs, as a great challenge for EA professionals, particularly those who have to operate the business, address the demands by current clients and customers and seek new customers. The challenge is identified in the lack of skills or poorly equipped professionals whose professional training and foundation have focused entirely on the development of clinical skills, not sales. These professionals often lack the skills and competencies required for the effective marketing of a product.

Marketing texts and writings have limited their attention and most of their examples to the marketing of goods. Another challenge when marketing EAPs is identified by Jenkins (2008) who stated that marketing a professional service like an EAP is very different from marketing a tangible product. The difficulty is associated with buyer anxieties and insecurities that can play a role in the purchasing decision-making process. The marketing strategy must therefore address the emotional and psychological concerns of potential buyers, which will be understood by studying the company's organizational culture and dynamics. This will ensure that the marketing strategy speaks directly to the needs of the client and addresses whatever concerns the company might have. Effective marketing of EAPs might change perceptions and certain buyer behaviors, which could impact on pricing.

The Marketing Environment

EAPs are operating in a complex environment. Internal and external factors seem to aggravate the complexity in pricing, in particular the processes involved in pricing that are sometimes known to the service providers but not to the corporate clients. It is important, therefore, that the marketer takes cognizance of the environmental influences within the market, which Marx and Van der Walt (1989) categorized as an environment that influences the relation between the marketer and the consumer. Such environmental factors potentially influence the marketing of a product or service (Marx & Van der Walt, 1989). Winegar (2002) highlighted the importance of defining the target market for EAP products. This target market is defined as potential customers who have a need, recognized or unrecognized, for EAP services. These potential customers also have the resources to purchase these EAP services.

Kawasaki (1995) argued that it is important to define and know one's customers. The authors have set out some questions that might guide service providers in gaining information about their customers:

- Who is using and who is buying your products?
  Acquiring information on who uses the product or service informs the service provider whether to refine the service or product to meet the demand.
- How do your customers use the products in your category?
  The service provider might discover that the assumptions that initially formed the basis for the service or product development are no longer relevant to meeting the customer's needs.
- Are laws, regulations or societal pressures changing your marketplace?
  In expanding the knowledge and understanding of the market in which EAPs operate, Winegar (2002) advised EAP professionals to use various ways of defining and segmenting markets for EAP services.

Buyer Behavior

Literature indicates that the marketing mix comprises the product, the price, the place/distribution, promotion, people, process, and physical environment/evidence. It is important, therefore, for marketers to consider the total marketing mix when setting prices (cf. Cowell, 1991; Jordaan & Prinsloo, 2001; Kotler & Armstrong, 2006; Winer, 2004).

In essence, this means that marketers must remember that customers rarely buy according to the price alone. They are looking for products that give them the best value in terms of the benefits received for the price paid. Ofir and Winer (2002) pointed out that when customers are confronted with a price or a set of prices, they process the price information and form preferences about the product service in question. Seeking the best value from the price paid and processing price information clearly indicates the price judgments made by customers when making purchasing decisions. Winer (2004) sensitized marketers to understanding and analyzing customer behavior when he identified five questions that must be addressed by marketers when designing a service or product:

- Who are the current and potential customers for the product or service?
- Why do they buy?
- How do they make purchasing decisions?
- Where do they buy the product/ services, that is, what channels of distribution are used?
- When do they buy?

With an understanding derived from the answers to these questions, EAP service providers will be in a position to tailor-make a service offering for each corporate client. This will ensure that the service offering meets the specific needs of the client to be served. Winer (2004) also emphasized the importance of analyzing competitors' customers, as this may go toward understanding why customers are buying one competitor's products instead of another. It is also important to analyze former customers. This means evaluation of the service offering, as this will help the service provider to understand weaknesses in their product of service operations. Answers to these questions might provide some ideas for stimulating brand-switching.

The State of Pricing in the EAP Field

Pricing is a challenge in the EAP field. Sharar and White (2001) perceived that the problem lies in the marketing of EAP services, which seem to be fuelled by deceptive marketing strategies for accumulating contracts. *Deception*, in this context, refers to the different ways in which sales representatives refrain from telling the truth about their products and services and slash their prices.

Such price slashing may lead to the submission of low bids by EAP service providers during tender processes.

Sharar and White (2001) further pointed out that price-slashing could lead to failure to conform to quality standards of service delivery, as clients would be channeled to less expensive telephonic interventions or even cheaper counseling sessions, despite the fact that their problems would require more sessions. Farris (2003) maintained that some of the complexities of the marketing environment in pricing are seen in instances where corporate clients individually engage in and negotiate the prices of products and services they want to procure. This complexity is a challenge to the EA professional to convince the purchaser that an EAP is not just another benefit but is rather a vital strategic partner that produces a significant return on investment, if properly promoted.

Kotler and Armstrong (2006) shared the view that pricing is the number one problem facing many marketing executives, leading to the improper handling of pricing. These authors support their assertion by identifying some of the common problems marketing executives encounter:

- Companies are too quick to reduce prices to get a sale rather than convincing buyers that their products are worth a higher price.
- Secondly, companies opt for pricing that is too cost oriented rather than consumer-value oriented.
- Lastly, companies look at pricing that does not take into consideration the rest of the marketing mix.

Doyle (2000) pointed out that difficulty with pricing seem to emanate from the accumulation of information that is inadequate to inform price decisions. To advance the notion of paying more for a quality service, Kotler and Armstrong (2006) argued that service providers should be in the position to persuade their customers that paying a high price for the required service is justified by the greater value it delivers. In other words, the value of the product is greater than the price tag.

Pricing of EAPS – the South African Experience

Standards for pricing EAPs, as laid out by the Standards Committee of EAPA-SA (2010), guide EAP practitioners, EAP service providers, and EAP corporate clients on how to adhere to these important guidelines. It is therefore important to know and understand the different pricing models used in the EAP field. Such knowledge and understanding form the basis on which to choose the best pricing model to meet the needs of the corporate client. Such information will also assist the corporate client in budgeting appropriately for the pricing model to be chosen for service provision. The Standards Committee of EAPA-SA stated that costing an EAP should be based on sound financial principles and should have the goal of ensuring the best application of financial resources. The objective is "to justify the balance between expenditure and benefits." It is important for the EAP service provider to explain all the different pricing models to give the corporate client the opportunity of making an informed decision. The Standards Committee of the EAPA-SA (p. 5) clearly outlined the criteria for costing models. These Standards state that the pricing of EAPs should be negotiated and mutually agreed upon by the service provider and the employer, after different models have been considered. The standard signifies the importance of corporate clients being conversant with pricing models.

The following types of pricing models are reflected in literature: capitated, pay for performance, utilization based, and value-based models (Attridge et al. 2010; Farris, 2003; Standards Committee of EAPA-SA, 2010). Special consideration should be given to the distinguishing characteristics of each model, with a clear understanding of the advantages and disadvantages. Subsequently, such an enhanced understanding will contribute toward making an informed decision on the choice of the pricing model that meets the needs of the corporate client.

METHOD

The objectives for this part of the study were to explore those factors that motivate corporate clients/consumers to choose or terminate the existing contract of a service provider, opting instead for another service provider. They should have the opportunity of exploring the internal and external constraints of the marketing environment that have an influence on the pricing of EAPs and that determine the choice of a specific EAP service delivery model. Finally they should be able to define a guideline for service providers that could be applied in practice as a standard EAP pricing model. Details on this last objective will, however, not be covered in this article, owing to space constraints, but will be submitted for publication separately.

A qualitative approach was adopted using the principles of applied research to bring about information that may help EAP service providers and corporate clients in decision-making processes about actual pricing, pricing models, and pricing processes used in the EAP field. Furthermore, the results of the research could possibly minimize some of the complexities associated with pricing in the EAP field.

Relative to the argument of understanding pricing in the EAP field, two groups of participants were targeted, participants from corporate clients who had terminated contracts with a leading EAP service provider, and staff members from this same leading EAP service provider. The rationale for two groups of participants is motivated by the complexities of pricing in the EAP field that would not be clearly understood if the focus was on one group only. The research population was comprised of five senior corporate well-being consultants from the leading EAP service provider. No sampling was done, as there were already only a limited number of available senior corporate well-being consultants. Two participants took part in the pilot study, data from which was not included in the final phase.

Regarding the corporate clients, the population was comprised of companies that had terminated contracts with a leading EAP service provider between 2007 and 2010. The participants were EAP coordinators and, in their absence, Human Resource (HR) managers and/or Procurement Department officers responsible for the tenders, EAP coordination, and termination of contracts. The sample size for this group of participants was based on the list of 30 company names of corporate clients obtained from the leading EAP service provider. There were challenges to accessing and getting permission from these companies. Some declined to participate in the study, with no clear reasons given, whereas others promised to come back to make appointments, which unfortunately they did not do. One of the researchers eventually interviewed five corporate clients.

The sampling method used in this part of the study (exploring information from the corporate clients) was purposive sampling, which is described as a type of sampling whereby the researchers select the units to be observed on the basis of own judgment as to which will be the most useful and representative (Babbie, 2004). To be specific, in the formulation and criteria used in choosing the units for the study, the authors focused on those participants who were responsible for acquiring new contracts, managing the accounts, renewing existing contracts, and terminating or closing existing contracts. The rationale for this criterion was based on the fact that these participants were confronted with the specifics and realities of pricing models based on the complexities involved in pricing.

A semistructured interview schedule was used as a data collection tool. Face-to-face interviews were conducted with participants to answer the research question: What are the complexities confronting a leading EAP service provider in South Africa regarding the pricing models used for pricing EAP services? Data was analyzed to develop themes and subthemes according to each question from the semistructured interview schedule. The identity of participants was subsequently protected.

FINDINGS

The range of participants' qualifications held by participants from the leading EAP service provider ranged through social work, psychology, law, and human resource management. The authors noted that a substantial number of participants had a background in social work. It is worth mentioning that few participants had pursued further studies in the EAP field, even by attending short courses on EAPs. This is significant to the study, because skills, expertise, and knowledge acquired through EAP short courses could contribute to the satisfaction of clients' needs. The marketing mix elements emphasize that training people is crucial if there are to be better results in marketing and delivery of quality service (Cowell, 1991; Jordaan & Prinsloo, 2001). Continued professional development or in-service training is crucial to ensuring that companies have the right people with the right attitudes and behavior to sustain good working relationships.

The majority of participants from corporate clients had studied human resource management. These participants viewed EAP as one of the HR benefits for its employees. It was also observed that these participants did not have much insight into the EAP field, except for counseling and seeing the program as a health awareness-raising tool. This finding demonstrates the danger associated with the appointment of an official without an EAP background. In essence, the official might be only an administrator, lacking the skill and expertise to interrogate the program against the standards set out by the Standards Committee of EAPA-SA (2010). When it comes to an understanding of the program design and implementation according to the set standards, the appointed person might lack expertise, as he or she might not have in-depth knowledge and understanding of EAPs.

Size of Companies and Nature of Business of Participating Corporate Clients

The corporate client sample was comprised of retail, financial, and government institutions. The findings revealed that financial businesses have a high number of employees whereas retail businesses have fewer. The size of the company and the nature of their business are significant when it comes to the design and implementation of the pricing model and results in a difference in approach to the choice of model. For instance, the findings indicate that the concern of the financial institutions about the well-being of their employees encourages them to search for the impact of EAP intervention. Their concern is driven by the fact that these employees are handling enormous financial sums, a responsibility that requires the well-being of the employees involved. The pricing model to be advocated for financial businesses must be comprehensive, addressing as many, if not all the risk factors that could affect these employees.

Results further revealed the importance of adjusting the reporting systems according to the specific need of the company served. This means that the reporting system must be discussed and agreed upon by the service provider and the corporate client. Of importance was the observation made about financial institutions who are concerned about the return of investment in terms of program outcomes. The reporting must therefore reflect the use and the value added by the program. For government institutions considerations should be given on red tape in relation to procurement processes that often affect the processes involved in the selection criteria and a choice of a pricing model. Furthermore, upon contracting considerations should be given on how to provide services to the diverse and extended families of the employee.

Qualitative Data According to Themes and Subthemes

COMPLEXITIES EXPERIENCED IN CONTRACTING FOR EAP SERVICES

Competition. The manner in which competition has unfolded in the EAP field seems to have encouraged price slashing among EAP service providers. On the other hand, competitive pricing seem to have encouraged corporate clients to find grounds for comparing prices among EAP service providers. The responses by participants from the leading EAP service provider in relation to competitors clearly indicate that competing solely on price seems to impact negatively on the adequate provision of services to corporate clients. Tough competition prompts other service providers to lower their prices, which at times results in services that do not necessarily fulfill the organizational needs of the corporate client.

Lee (2005) confirmed the above findings, stating that the EAP environment has become so competitive that prices, which were too low to start with, have not increased sufficiently in years, making it difficult to provide services and to survive. The author further indicated that a low price prompts EAP service providers to give as little service as possible. Hartley (2006), on the other hand, maintained that EAPs worldwide seem to compete primarily on the basis of price, although there may be referral to advantages like superior quality or responsiveness during the bidding process. Price, as the basis for competition, has led to the predictable result that there is slow but steady pressure for EAP service providers to do more for less.

The study conducted by Burke and Sharar (2009) presented views on the complexity of the competition in the EAP field, where the EAP marketplace is identified as extremely competitive, with EAP providers continually lowering prices to retain business. There is pressure on EAP providers to lower prices whereas service expectations from clients remain the same or increase, creating an untenable dilemma for EAP providers. This results in sacrifices being made by service providers in terms of profit margins to retain contracts.

The results reflect that the EAP service providers in South Africa are also under pressure to deliver more quality services at minimal cost owing to corporate clients' resistance to price increases. The responses from corporate clients indicate that service providers compete primarily on prices to ensure that business is retained, but with little difference in the service offering.

Price. The responses shared by corporate clients who believed that EAP services are fairly priced seem to express belief in the quality of services rendered and the value of such services. The relationship between price and perceived quality service is also highlighted by Burke (2008), who mentioned that purchasers generally expect to pay an appropriate price for quality. The authors support this view with research findings which show that a high price is perceived to equate with high quality, whereas a low price means low quality. This view, however, is disputed by participants from a leading EAP service provider, whose rationale for low pricing is based on a strategic decision to obtain a contract without compromising the quality of the service.

The results indicate the difficulty of setting a right price that adequately meets the comprehensive service offering. The challenges seem to emanate from price sensitivity, which tends to force service providers to lower their prices. Maynard (2003) mentioned that EAPs have been caught in a deflationary spiral of decreasing prices, whereas pricing affects everything conducted by EAPs, including service offering. The inability to charge reasonable prices for EAP services affects the quality of the programs, livelihoods, and professional esteem, and ultimately the survival of the EAP as a viable concept. Jenkins (2008) seemed to associate price challenges with pricing wars that compromise quality servicing, putting companies in the position of charging less, whereas overhead costs are increasing. In this study, the results indicate that price wars have negative repercussions on the corporate client and the EAP service provider. Unfortunately, the implications of service limitations and exclusions seem not to be seriously considered during contracting until clients are confronted with the realities of low pricing.

Sharar and Hertenstein (2006) maintained that the greatest challenge facing the EAP field is finding avenues to help HR professionals and benefits for managers to understand and appreciate the potential of an effective EAP, as well as to overcome low expectations of what an EAP can accomplish. The challenge identified is that most purchasers are not in a position to understand that an EAP can be overpriced, depending on the outcomes the EAP achieves.

The responses echoed by the participants from corporate clients indicated that the cheapest bid is not always the best in terms of service offering. However, senior managers require a lot of convincing before they contract with a service provider who puts out the highest bid. Jenkins (2008) stated that there has been a failure to clearly and factually educate senior leadership on the value of EAP as an organizational assistance tool, as opposed to simply being a behavioral healthcare benefit.

Different pricing models. Another pricing challenge in the EAP field is the lack of uniform standards for the pricing of EAP services. The challenge is identified in the comment made by a corporate client that there was no benchmark in terms of pricing models used in the EAP field. The statement indicated that EAP service providers seem to decide on their own standard for pricing, which causes confusion for corporate clients, who are confronted with highly competitive prices from EAP service providers. The lack of standard practice in pricing is also seen in the attempts used by service providers to come up with their own benchmarks in terms of price increase. Sharar and Hertenstein (2006) identified three primary reforms that would enable the EAP field to break free from the commodity price-driven market. First, purchasers and EA professionals should be educated in selling and buying on the basis of compliance with quality standards rather than the lowest price. Second, the EAP field should conduct conclusive, evidence-based research comparing the effect of various EAP models and the costs of these models on productivity losses and treatment outcomes. Last, there should be design and implementation of new pricing schemes that blend elements of the capitation model and fee for service with meaningful performance guarantees and risk sharing. It is important, therefore, to have some standard guidelines for practice which include a regulatory framework for the fee structure.

The results indicate a gap in the sharing of information on the different pricing models by a leading EAP service provider. Corporate clients seem to take what is offered to them without necessarily providing options. On the other hand, corporate clients, especially those responsible for contracting and management of EAP within the company, do not educate themselves about pricing models. Corporate clients ought to know about the different pricing models to choose the most suitable pricing model to meet their organization's needs. Popular approaches to the pricing of EAP services include the capitated model, which is the most common, the utilization-based model, the "pay-for-performance" model and value-based models. Each of these models has its merits and its concerns. It becomes important to advise purchasers of EAP services to consider which kind of pricing model is most likely to create the business incentives that match the goals of the EAP (Attridge, et al., 2010; Farris, 2003; Standards Committee of EAPA-SA, 2010).

The advantage of engaging service providers for different pricing models was shared by one corporate client who approached service providers for proposals other than the tender process. This allowed an opportunity for the corporate client to identify the preferred suitable pricing model. It was interesting to note that the service provider advocated for the capitated model with motivations that were not welcomed by the corporate client. The negotiation process culminated in the choice of a combined model.

It is clear that knowledge of the different pricing models and procedures on how prices are calculated minimized corporate clients' lack of understanding of the costs of EAP services. This was identified as a gap by participants from a leading EAP service provider. Knowledge of the different pricing models and sharing of such information with corporate clients is important and is in line with one of the criteria for costing models, as outlined by the Standards Committee of EAPA-SA (2010). The standard states that the pricing of EAPs should be negotiated and mutually agreed upon by the service provider and the employer, after different models have been considered. These findings relating to knowledge about the different pricing models lead us to the discussion on transparency of the pricing models in the EAP field.

From the findings on transparency relating to pricing models and the cost of EAP service, it is evident that the pricing, marketing, selling, and buying of professional services is a complex process. Such complexity is owing to the intangible nature of these services, whose value is at times not immediate in comparison with the value of goods. The result is therefore the inability of a leading EAP service provider to share certain costs with corporate clients.

It is important for corporate clients to take into consideration the fact that the EAP is actually a prepaid service for unforeseen circumstances. The availability of services therefore means that a service provider is constantly available to address the clients' needs. This is expensive, as counselors have to be readily available should a crisis occur. However, this view should not be seen in the light of the EAP as a reactionary service, seeing that there are other services that are proactive in nature. The costs should be clearly defined upfront. Bradman (2003) mentioned that it is high time for EAPs to remove the smoke and mirrors atmosphere that currently pervades EAP pricing. The authors advise that EAPs adopt comprehensive disclosure policies that will accurately represent the pricing bases for EAP services. The authors further advise that such a disclosure would allow purchasers to compare similar attributes when purchasing EAP services.

Part of this theme on pricing models was supported by EAPA-SA in relation to costing models that are currently being contravened, as service providers continue to follow the trend of underpricing. It was important, therefore, to present recommendations on how the EAP field could overcome the issue of noncompliance with EAPA-SA standards in relation to costing models. There would also have to be a recommendation on how the EAP field could ensure that the EAP remained relevant in a competitive and complex environment confronted by challenges in contracting.

The responses of participants from a leading EAP service provider pointed out that corporate clients have encouraged the bidding war with their selection criteria in tender processes. On the other hand, corporate clients believe the service offerings from EAP service providers are the same, making it difficult for them to choose which service provider to contract with. Price thus becomes the differentiating factor. Comments made indicated that there was a great challenge facing EAP service providers in terms of what determines appropriate pricing, taking into consideration the input variables, which differ from one service provider to another. It becomes a challenge when getting to the practical implementation of the standard of costing models as set out by the Standards Committee of EAPA-SA (2010), which states that costing EAPs should be based on sound financial principles, with the goal of ensuring the best application of financial resources. The objective, which is "to justify the balance between expenditure and benefits," seems difficult to measure, as participants, particularly those from corporate clients, seem to find difficulty in justifying to their executives the balance between expenditure and the benefits of the program. Participants from the financial sector linked the challenge to the reporting mechanisms whereby service providers' reports do not speak business language in terms of the return on investment as well as the monies that a company invests in the EAP.

This inability to speak in terms of business requires EAP service providers and corporate clients to seriously consider exactly what these sound financial principles with which they must comply are when costing EAPs. Furthermore, the pricing model must take into consideration the costs of the quality service offering, where quality must be prioritized. Once again, the challenges posed by tender procedures minimize the opportunity for meaningful engagement between corporate clients and service providers. The challenge can be identified in the situation wherein the tender process encourages service providers to prepack service offerings, and decide for the corporate client what will be offered, without necessarily providing an open and transparent process of engagement. Currently there are fixed prices for service offerings. Only in negotiations may one have the opportunity to cut down on services that are deemed unnecessary and pay only for what is necessary and should be available for employees.

Contracting. The responses by the participants from a leading EAP service provider in relation to price variation in contracting indicate that clients' circumstances are taken into consideration when pricing is done. It is the authors' opinion that such consideration given to clients may result in the pricing process becoming subjective in nature and may therefore raise questions of objectivity in pricing in the EAP field.

The process of comparing prices is complex, because comparison is subjective and perceptual in nature. The subjective nature of price comparison is associated with the criteria used by corporate clients to compare one service provider with another, and likewise such criteria vary from one corporate client to another. The subjective nature of price comparison is reiterated by a substantial number of participants from a leading EAP service provider, who maintained that the pricing model used by their company is very competitive. As a result, most of the clients contract with them. However, when corporate clients decide to terminate a contract, choosing instead a low-priced service provider, it raises questions about which services are being compromised by the competing service provider.

Buyer behavior has a major influence on contracting. Purchasers such as EAP service providers must understand consumer behavior. Marx and Van der Walt (1989) maintained that understanding consumer decision making is the most crucial aspect of marketing management. Weitz and Wensely (2002) expanded on this view of buyer behavior and subjectivity regarding price, mentioning that many customers actively process price information, which means that they are not just price takers. Buyers continually assess the price charged for products according to prior purchasing experience. The information on the criteria used to select and contract with EAP service providers shared by the majority of participants from corporate clients, and the cost of the service and the value attached, which is informed by met or unmet expectations from previous contracts, came out strongly. Eventually these considerations become a deciding factor in a contract.

Economy. Historically, EAPs were founded on the assumption that there would be economic gains for companies through increasing productivity. However, the decline in the global economy threatens the comprehensive provision of EAP services. The participants from a leading EAP service provider's responses show clearly that EAPs seem to be under threat of elimination or of facing budget cuts when companies are confronted with financial difficulties. The researchers maintain that the underlying reasons for this action are still uncertain, as it seems to contradict the original view held of EAPs. The dual benefit of having an EAP in the work organizations is demonstrated in the description of EAP provided by Gornick and Blair (2005) and Pilette (2005), whose views are embedded in the utilization of specific core technologies to enhance employee and workplace effectiveness, thereby making business sense for the organization. The researchers maintain that, to make these benefits known, EAPs have to undertake a number of processes. Kim (1988) identified program evaluation as a significant process that provides vital information on the need, implementation, and impact of the program. Economic efficiency, which is the tangible way of calculating the program in terms of cost benefit or cost effectiveness analysis, is identified as crucial if EAPs are to survive budget cuts during difficult economic times. To emphasize the position and possible gains of EAPs for work organizations, Maiden (1988) argued that EAPs must demonstrate their economic effectiveness and cost-efficiency to remain a viable part of the organization rather than becoming a financial drain for which there is no return on investment.

In the analysis of the findings on the impact of the economy on EAPs, being informed about the historic view of EAPs and their historical economic benefit to companies, the researchers have concerns as to why EAPs are now first in line for budget cuts when companies experience financial difficulties. The finding raises questions about the perceptions and views held on EAPs by HR and executive managers. The researchers argue that answers to these questions could be provided by further research into return on investment, when scientific findings should be presented to build a stronger case for EAP pricing. Currently, minimal research on return on investment is conducted. This gap in research seems to prompt questions by companies on gains presented by EAPs. For this reason, questions are raised when annual price increases are proposed in relation to contract renewals. On the other hand, EAP service providers submit low bids to obtain and sustain contracts.

Internal processes in preparation for submission of a bid for a contract. The research findings indicate that a number of factors are considered and processes are undertaken in preparation for a bid. These factors and processes require EAP service providers to conduct organizational profiling and assessment to understand the needs of the company to be served. The identified factors in this study are the company's budget, the size of the company, utilization, the service offering, the relationship with the client, and the input factors considered in pricing.

Company's budget. The participants from a leading EAP service provider's responses indicate that a company's budget allocation plays a crucial role in the choice of a pricing model. The results seem to indicate that there is no adherence to EAPA-SA standards and guidelines for practice in relation to budget allocation for EAPs. When participants indicated that some companies did not prioritize EAPs when budgeting, this raised the researchers' concern, as clear guidelines are stipulated by the Standards Committee of EAPA-SA (2010) in relation to the costing of EAP services. The Committee mentioned states that a comprehensive budget should be compiled in alignment with the organizational budget. The guidelines should therefore guide budget allocation for EAPs. Possible reasons for the lack of adherence could be that companies are not conversant with these standards and guidelines for practice when setting up an EAP in their company.

The finding implies that companies should have a clear understanding of organizational needs to allocate a satisfactory budget for EAPs. Budget allocation should be informed by the knowledge of possible pricing models to ensure the provision of a comprehensive service package for the organization. The problem of proper budget allocation for EAPs is identified by Burke and Sharar (2009), who stated that EAPs are a low-profile program and a low-budget priority. This implies that it is therefore easy to cut the EAP budget or even allocate insufficient resources for program implementation.

The other finding that stood out in the study in relation to budget was the lack of budget disclosure by some corporate clients. The researchers maintain that lack of disclosure hinders the process of selecting an appropriate pricing model by service providers to ensure that the needs of corporate clients are met. Budget disclosure enables the service provider to discuss openly with the corporate client the services that could be offered on the available budget. Disclosure further provides an opportunity for the service provider to tailor-make services that would accommodate the client's available budget. The service provider is also in a better position to further advise the corporate client (in cases of contract renewal) on how the program would shrink from the original services that were provided for in the initial contract.

Size of the company. Taking into consideration the size of the company and the cost implications, the results indicate that there are varying degrees of expectation between large and small companies in relation to the cost implications of EAP pricing models. Burke and Sharar (2009) stated that, though small companies are more likely to embed or opt for low cost EAP, owing to limitations in their financial and human resources, their decision to have an EAP will be cost driven, while they also appreciate its value. Larger employers consider economics, while their driving force is the value added. Govender (2009) alluded to the size of an organization's work-force as a critical factor in the decision to have an EAP.

Utilization. Utilization is considered an important variable in the choice of a pricing model. Responses from service providers and corporate clients indicate a level of uncertainty as to how this important variable could best be calculated and presented. Literature indicates that reporting utilization is quite a complex issue, as confirmed by Hartley (2006) when pointing out that the EAP industry lacks uniformity on how to measure and report on EAP services. Sharar and Masi (2006) expanded on the problem of calculating utilization rates, stating that, though there are no agreed-upon or standard definitions for calculating utilization rates, utilization reports are submitted to employers without indicating how the numbers were derived. Subsequently, the lack of uniformity and clarity on how to measure utilization reduces to assumptions decisions about employers' performance. The complexity comes with the difficulty of what should be included in reporting on utilization and how this should be done. Jorgensen and Brooks (2007) stated that the EAP industry has fallen into the trap of trying to communicate value simply by virtue of utilization and whoever produces the highest numbers at the lowest cost wins. Unfortunately this has not demonstrated value to companies, as it does not communicate what is done by EAPs in real terms, in a format that employers and HR managers will understand, respect, appreciate and want. The authors take the discussion further, pointing out that the problem lies in the reporting tools used by EAPs, when many of their reporting tools have not adequately met business reporting and communication demands (Jorgensen, 2007).

Participants from a leading EAP service provider indicated that, when a pricing model such as capitation is based on the estimated utilization rate and few clients utilize the service, there is no refund for underutilization. However, if the client overutilizes the service, an additional fee is charged. In circumstances where the client uses the service fully within the contracted budget, that becomes a win-win situation for both the service provider and the corporate client.

This finding points out the discrepancies experienced with utilization. The results indicate that, if EAPs want to make a strong business case, they should help those who purchase EAP services to make the link between EAP activities and business needs by formulating comprehensive and well-conceptualized reports.

Service offering (type of services). Responses from the EAP service provider and the corporate clients by participants indicate the importance of offering a comprehensive basket of services. This indicates that service providers must be clear as to the mode of service offering (in this instance, face-to-face or telephonic), as the "how" aspect determines how costly the service will be. The evaluation of service offerings for existing contracts considered for renewal was identified as significant. Yamatani (1993) called this evaluation program adequacy assessment, as it examines the appropriateness of EAP in terms of service availability, usage, and penetration rates. Service evaluation provides an opportunity to identify service gaps. It also provides an opportunity for the service provider and the corporate client to review the pricing model and determine whether it still meets the needs of the company. The results of the findings indicate that corporate clients' evaluation of service offering during the evaluation of bids is informed by the experiences of service offerings by previously contracted service providers.

The delivery of quality service that adds value to the company is the significant determinant, and failure to demonstrate these variables puts EAP service providers at risk of losing contracts. Nonetheless, how to evaluate these determinants is problematic unless measures are put in place in the contracting phase. In professional services the quality standards and value-added are subjective matters that will be determined by the recipient of the service.

Relationship with the corporate client. The relationship between the service provider and corporate clients is crucial in the EAP field and such relationships must be perceived positively by both parties. The responses from data provided by the majority of participants from a leading EAP service provider indicate that if relationships are perceived negatively it is likely to affect the renewal of a contract. Positive relationships are those characterized by trust, honesty and openness and should go hand-in-hand with transparency in the pricing models used by EAP service providers.

Terblanche (2010) confirmed the importance of communication for the successful contracting of a costing model, a view that was shared by corporate clients.

Embedded costs. Responses from a leading EAP service provider indicate that certain costs are difficult to explain when contracting with corporate clients. The difficulty stems from the inability to account for such costs, and yet the client has paid or is required to pay. Although participants from a leading EAP service provider identify the difficulty to explain certain costs to corporate clients, the authors argue that sharing information on costs displays the level of transparency. Transparency enables corporate clients to clearly understand what goes into the pricing models and might minimize the challenges and questions that are often raised when a price increase is proposed. Bradman (2003) emphasized that there are many factors to be considered in arriving at an appropriate capitation rate, including prior usage, administrative expenses, payments to providers, case management costs, outsourcing costs, reserves, and profits. Therefore capitation as a statistical and actuarial tool should be transparent about the costs involved in the pricing models used by EAP service providers.

Role players involved in the contracting process and their impact. The responses by a leading EAP service provider indicate that an extensive consultation process is carried out by a leading EAP service provider when compiling a proposal for a bid. Corporate clients also engage in a similar process to get a buy-in by internal stakeholders before the final decision is taken to contract a particular service provider. Data presented by the leading EAP service provider and corporate clients indicates the influence of the different stakeholders on the decision-making process. The perceptions held by different role players regarding service offering and the EAP as a whole might impact on the resource allocations and might subsequently affect the choice of a pricing model.

In emphasizing the impact of other role players on EAPs when contracting, Carbone (2003) stated that most managers, HR professionals, and chief financial officers are under pressure to show a return on investment for every program they sponsor, despite the slow economy. It therefore becomes significant for EAPs to prove to business leaders and other role players who decide on contracting the value of the service that has been provided (in the case of renewal) and the service to be provided (in the case of a new contract).

The findings indicate that the internal role players, such as business units from a leading EAP service provider, are experts in their respective fields. They are knowledgeable about service offering, the required resources, and the costs of rendering such services. These role players have expert knowledge of the EAP, so their input is important and contributes toward the overall pricing model to be advocated to the corporate client.

In a comparison of role players from a leading EAP service provider with those of corporate clients, the latter are seen to have a combination of different role players. Some are not necessarily knowledgeable about the EAP, and their main interest is in seeing the balance between cost and perceived or expected benefit and results (Lennox, Sharar, & Burke, 2009). The researchers identified the importance of educating these role players to curb one of the dilemmas facing the EAP field when selling EAP. Fauria (2009) stated that EAP purchasers are not sufficiently informed to be able to distinguish different EAP models, so their decision making during contracting is based on price.

The inclusion of business units by corporate clients during the consultation process for evaluation of a proposal is seen as significant. The involvement of business units presents an opportunity to gain a holistic picture of employees' needs, and to ensure that the inputs of business units are taken into consideration in the evaluation of proposals. The authors maintain that the involvement of these stakeholders and their opinions might have a significant impact on deciding which pricing model will offer better services to meet the employees' needs. Their involvement might create a sense of ownership of the program, including its utilization should their input in contracting be taken into consideration.

EXTERNAL PROCESSES ENCOUNTERED IN THE SUBMISSION OF A BID AND CONTRACT RENEWAL

Procurement procedures for professional services. A view shared by corporate clients within government sector indicates that the procurement procedure and the processes currently followed by supply chain management, where the lowest bid wins, affect negatively the selection of service providers and contracting with them. The negative repercussion can be seen when contracting with a service provider who has no credibility or track record of service offering in the EAP field. The result means contracting with inexperienced service providers just to comply with procurement procedures. The credibility of service providers with a good service record in terms of delivering quality work is one of the main elements considered in the selection criteria for contracting. Sharar and Hertenstein (2006) identified the problem with procurement procedures as a process that seems to have encouraged service providers to bid low. These authors point out that the "lowest price bid game" seems "to be endemic and widespread in the procurement process, fueling a type of rhetorical marketing competition among EAP vendors themselves." One of the participants from a leading EAP service provider shared their own experience of being very cautious during the briefing meeting for bidding. The participant carefully selected words during briefing sessions not to expose or reveal too much about the bidder's own company. The authors are of the opinion that assumptions made might lead to the submission of unrealistic bids.

Quality of services. The study undertaken by Jenkins (2008) concurs with the experiences encountered by the corporate client in relation to a low bid and quality of service. The author found that "EAPs are so focused on survival in a very tight and increasingly competitive marketplace that the drive to reduce costs of operation is affecting the delivery of services to the organization and the employee" (p. 42).

In this study, the result of findings indicated that service providers in South Africa are also under pressure to deliver quality services, while they are confronted with the challenge of corporate clients who are price sensitive and often use price as a criterion in contracting. It is important for EAP service providers to strive for the delivery of quality service in the midst of unhealthy competition instead of lowering prices, which could subsequently have a negative impact on providing comprehensive services that meet the expectations of a client's organization.

Selection criteria. The results also revealed that the criteria used by corporate clients are their expectations, which are measured against their previous experiences of contracting with earlier service providers. Some corporate clients were not entirely clear about either their expectations or the services required. Their discovery of other services was made with the evaluation process of proposal, when some service providers put add-ons into their service offerings. Such services are presented as free of charge, and the corporate client suddenly realizes they would benefit from such services. Such corporate clients therefore select and contract with the other service provider on the basis of free additional services. The action raises concern about the selection criteria used by corporate clients and seems to indicate a lack of adherence to bidding specifications and clear criteria used for selection.

KEY RECOMMENDATIONS

- EAP service providers must make an effort to educate the corporate client about the different pricing models, explaining the advantages and disadvantages of each model.
- EAP service providers must be more transparent about the costs involved in a pricing model.
- Corporate clients must also take the responsibility of empowering themselves with information on the different pricing models. Coupled with such understanding, corporate clients must conduct an organizational

profile, including the needs assessment for the organization to ensure that an informed decision is made on selecting a best pricing model to meet organizational needs.

- The EAP field must have a standard practice of pre- and postevaluations of the state of the organization in relation to the utilization of EAP services because the results of interventions are observed over a period of time.
- Utilization must be calculated, interpreted, and presented in a well-developed and recognized reporting manner agreed upon by the service provider and the corporate client.
- There must be education on EAP services and their value to all the levels of management, including executive managers. Education and information sharing should put emphasis on budget allocation for EAP services and alignment of the EAP budget with the EAP policies developed to guide their implementation through the utilization of acknowledged guidelines, that is, EAPA-SA EAP standards and comparable documentation from other countries like the United States, the United Kingdom, and Australia.
- EAP policies and strategies must be effectively implemented, with full support from executive management.
- Training in customer care also becomes significant, as relationships are a determinant in sustaining contracts.
- Service providers should strive to build their credibility through intensive processes in the selection and training of line functionaries who represents the image of the company.
- Quality in service offering must be prioritized by the EAP service providers, as the study revealed that the provision of sustainable quality service is achieved through appropriate pricing and allocation of resources. Corporate clients must therefore be prepared to reward the provision of quality services.
- Corporate clients must be more transparent when it comes to the criteria for the selection of a service provider. Selection based on the lowest bid (price) must be avoided.
- Corporate clients must influence a paradigm shift in low bidding by strengthening transparent and consistent selection criteria that do not prioritize price as a deciding factor.
- EAP service providers must understand buyer behavior and incorporate such understanding into the marketing strategy. Marketing must focus on the value attached to the program based on testimonials and success stories on best practices.
- There must be clear service-level agreements signed by both parties to optimize transparency, honesty, and respect for the contractual obligation from both parties i.e., the corporate client and the service provider. Such service-level agreements will ensure that corporate clients' expectations are met.
- Flexibility in service offering must be considered after both parties have explored, negotiated, and agreed on all the available options, such as

restructuring of the service package or even payment for additional services not covered within the contractual obligation.

- Corporate clients must conduct comprehensive organizational profiling and clearly articulate what they want to make available to their employees. Clear expectations will provide an opportunity for bidding service providers to present their business case and engage with the prospective corporate client.

CONCLUSION

The research study gathered valuable data on what participants from a leading EAP service provider and corporate clients who had terminated contracts perceived to be standard practices that should apply in the EAP field. The study revealed deficiencies relating to scientific data that would justify costs for EAP services. These deficiencies, such as lack of benchmarks in pricing and reporting on utilization, continue to cause discrepancies in motivations to pay more for EAP services.

The researchers developed guidelines that could be applied as standard practice for EAP pricing models to be published at a later stage. It is important to note in this study that EAPs are encouraged to achieve the best results by promoting the provision of quality programs and not simply judging according to price. The quality of programs should be judged on program results which will be measured through outcomes for employees and the work organization. Emphasis is placed on corporate clients to consider several factors to determine the quality and value of the program when contracting with service providers.

REFERENCES

Attridge, M. (2007). Answering 10 questions. *Journal of Employee Assistance, 37*(3), 27–30.

Attridge, M., Amaral, T., Bjornson, T., Goplerud, E., Herlihy, P., McPherson, T., ... Teems, L. (2010). Pricing options for EAP services. *EASNA Research Notes, 1*(6), 1–3.

Babbie, E. (2004). *The practice of social research* (10th ed.). Belmont, CA: Wadsworth/Thomson Learning.

Bradman, L. H. (2003). Apples to apples. *Journal of Employee Assistance, 4*, 7.

Burke, J. (2008). The lessons of free EAPs. *Journal of Employee Assistance, 38*(2), 17–18.

Burke, J., & Sharar, D. A. (2009). Do free EAPs offer a discernible value? *Journal of Employee Assistance, 39*(3), 6–9.

Carbone, J. (2003, June). Use everyday examples to prove your value: Providing specific examples of money-saving risk management services can help EAPs prove they are worth premium rates. *Journal of Employee Assistance, 33*(2), 22–23.

Cowell, D. W. (1991). *The marketing of services*. Stoneham, MA: Butterworth-Heinemann.

Doyle, P. (2000). *Value based marketing. Marketing strategies for corporate growth and shareholder value*. Chichester, UK: Wiley & Sons.

Fauria, T. M. (2009). Commodity or craft: The choice is ours. *Journal of Employee Assistance, 39*(3), 13–15.

Farris, T. (2003, June). A new approach to EAP pricing: value-based pricing models create incentives for EAPs to increase utilization and help employers understand the benefits EAPs provide. *The Journal of Employee Assistance, 33*(2), 24–26.

Gornick, M. E., & Blair, B. R. (2005). Employee assistance, work-life effectiveness, health and productivity: A conceptual framework for integration. In M. Attridge, P. A. Herlihy, & R. P. Maiden (Eds.), *The integration of employee assistance, work/life and wellness services* (pp. 1–29). New York, NY: Haworth Press.

Govender, T. (2009). *A critical analysis of the prevalence and nature of the employee assistance program in the Eastern Cape Buffalo City Municipal Area* (Unpublished masters' thesis). University of Pretoria, Pretoria, South Africa.

Hartley, M. (2006). Competing on higher ground: Marketing of Employee Assistance Programs. *Journal of Employee Assistance, 36*(1), 4.

Jenkins, R. S. (2008). *The Employee Assistance Program management yearbook* (3rd ed.). Manasquan, NJ: American Business Publishing.

Jordaan, Y., & Prinsloo, M. (2001). *Grasping service marketing*. Pretoria, South Africa: Grapevine News.

Jorgensen, D. G. (2007). Demonstrating EAP value. *Journal of Employee Assistance, 37*(3), 24–26.

Jorgensen, D., & Brooks, R. (2007). Demonstrating EAP value: Preaching what we practice. *Journal of Employee Assistance, 37*(1), 16–17.

Kawasaki, G. (1995). *How to drive your competition crazy: Creating disruption for fun and profit*. New York, NY: Hyperion.

Kim, D. S. (1988). Assessing Employee Assistance Programs. In M. J. Holosko & M. D. Feit (Eds.), *Evaluation of Employee Assistance Program* (pp. 169–185). New York, NY: Haworth Press.

Kotler, P., & Armstrong, G. (2006). *Principles of marketing* (11th ed.). Upper Saddle River, NJ: Pearson Prentice Hall.

Lee, K. (2005). Low prices drag EAP quality down. *Employee Benefit News, 19*(1), 1–40.

Lennox, R., Sharar, D., & Burke, J. (2009). Measuring workplace outcomes in EAPs: Until EAPs can demonstrate they produce positive workplace outcomes, they will continue to lack credibility with employers and be seen as commodities. *The Journal of Employee Assistance, 39*(4), 18.

Maiden, R. P. (1988). Employee Assistance Program evaluation in a federal government agency. In M. J. Holosko & M. D. Feit (Eds.), *Evaluation of Employee Assistance Programs* (pp. 191–202). New York, NY: Haworth Press.

Marx, S., & Van der Walt, A. (1989). *Marketing management*. Cape Town, South Africa: Juta & Co, Ltd.

Maynard, J. (2003). The market doesn't drive pricing – we do. *Journal of Employee Assistance, 33*(2), 2.

Ofir, C., & Winer, R. (2002). Pricing: Economic and behavioural models. In B. Weitz & R. Wensely (Eds.), *Handbook of marketing* (pp. 267–281). London, UK: Sage.

Peters, H. J. (1999). A value-driven approach to the operations of a South African EAP vendor. *Employee Assistance Quarterly, 14*(3), 83–84.

Pilette, P. C. (2005, Winter). EAPs are good investments for managing presenteeism. *EAP Digest*, 17–19.

Sharar, D. (2004, May 31). With HR chasing lowest prices, EAPs can't improve quality. *Canadian HR Reporter, 17*(11), 6–7.

Sharar, D., & Hertenstein, E. (2006). Perspectives on commodity pricing in Employee Assistance Programs (EAPs): A survey of the EAP field. *World at Work Journal, 5*(1), 32–41.

Sharar, D., & Masi, D. A. (2006). Crises facing the EAP field. *Journal of Employee Assistance, 36*(4), 7–9.

Sharar, D., & White, W. (2001, Fall). EAP ethics and quality. *EAP Digest*, 16–19.

Standards Committee of Employee Assistance Professionals Association of South Africa (EAPA-SA). (2010). *Standards of Employee Assistance Programs in South Africa*. Unpublished report. Pretoria, South Africa.

Terblanche, L. S. (2010, October 8). *Benchmarking clients' expectations against providers' product*. Paper presented at an EAP international conference, Tampa, FL.

Weitz, B., & Wensely, R. (2002). *Handbook of marketing*. London, UK: Sage.

Winegar, N. (2002). *Employee Assistance Programs in managed care: Marketing and selling EAPs*. New York, NY: Haworth Press.

Winer, R. S. (2004). *Marketing management* (2nd ed.). Upper Saddle River, NJ: Prentice Hall.

Yamatani, H. (1993). Suggested top ten evaluations for Employee Assistance Programs: An overview. *Employee Assistance Quarterly, 9*(2), 65–82.

The Effects of Psychosocial Problems on Employees' Stress, Self-Esteem, and Organizational Commitment: The Case of South Korean Workplaces

SOOCHAN CHOI, MSW, PhD

School of Social Welfare, Yonsei University, Seoul, South Korea

JEONGEUN LEE, MSW, PhD

Department of Rehabilitation Medicine, Seoul National University Hospital, Seoul, South Korea

HAEWOONG PARK, MSW, PhD

Korea Expressway Corporation, Seoul, South Korea

The psychosocial problems that today's employees are facing can cause considerable stress, and such stress is likely to affect negatively their individual traits as well as organizational fulfillment. This study thus analyzed the impacts of the employees' psychosocial problems, which occurred widely in work life, family life, and cultural- and health-related life, on their stress, self-esteem, and organizational commitment. Seven hundred and thirty employees in a public enterprise in South Korea were randomly selected, and the research method of the structural equation model with survey questionnaires was applied. The results of the study confirmed that the psychosocial problems that the workers have confronted influenced stress, which was proved to deteriorate their level of organizational commitment and their self-esteem. This implies that more systematic assistance and management of the psychosocial problems must be developed.

Today people working for companies are forced to confront various difficulties, such as heavy workloads, severe competition with colleagues, and the high risk of unemployment. They also find it difficult to deal with personal issues, such as child-rearing, caring for elderly parents, and marital conflicts all of which must affect their occupational lives (Myers, 1984). The problems that the workers encounter in their work and family lives are likely to prompt psychosocial difficulties such as stress, depression, anxiety, and low self-esteem. Furthermore, these problems often cause absenteeism, frequent employee turnover, and low levels of organizational commitment and job performance (Latack, 1984).

However, individual psychosocial problems do relate to workers' social environments. Sophisticatedly designed social support structures will reduce workers' psychosocial problems, whereas inefficient or insufficient social support may not alleviate these problems at all (House, 1981). Personal social networks are often volatile and do not comprise the resources necessary to overcome psychosocial problems. Thus, many work organizations have developed Employee Assistance Programs (EAPs) to intervene in and prevent employees' psychosocial problems. EAPs are currently prevalent in most developed countries, and their performance has been deemed effective in most previous studies (Kelly, Holbrook, & Bragen, 2005; U.S. Department of Labor, 1990). However, Korean companies still have few systematic supporting service systems like EAPs, even though they are in great need by workers suffering from psychosocial problems (Choi, 2006).

This study therefore focuses on employees' psychosocial problems and analyzes their impacts at individual and organizational levels. In particular, it examines the effects of employees' psychological problems on their stress, self-esteem, and their commitment to the organizations they belong to. This research aims throughout to identify efficient and practical workers' support systems and to provide grounds for activating the practical services needed to reestablish employees' mental health and organizational validity.

BACKGROUND

Workers' Psychosocial Problems and Stress

Companies expect their employees to deal with heavy workloads to survive the relentless global competition existing today. However, such expectations often cause a range of accompanying difficulties for their employees. In particular, most employees in South Korea are facing unstable employment due to unpredictable lay-offs since the economic crisis of the late 1990s—heavy workloads, severe competition within their own company, and maladjustment to organizations—all of which lead to high levels of stress and psychogenic diseases (Burke, 1991; Chang, 2002; Voydanoff, 1989).

Family problems also tend to affect occupational lives, causing work–family conflicts and, accordingly, a significant level of stress for workers (Carlson, Kacmar, & Williams, 2000; Paik & Choi, 2006). Indeed, family and work cannot realistically be considered independently, and changes to one part inevitably prompt changes to the other (Voydanoff, 1989). Today, as 60% of the women in South Korea participate in the workforce, more and more married couples are suffering from the difficulty of contending with the care of elderly parents, their children's education, marital conflicts, and family separation (McCroskey & Scharlach, 1993; Paik & Choi, 2006). Caring for elderly parents, rearing children, and heavy household chores are likely to reduce employees' working hours and hamper employees in their duties and commitment to their companies.

Finally, employees in South Korea tend to encounter a variety of stress-causing health and medical issues. Alcohol problems, smoking, and diet-related problems are threatening workers' physical and mental health that, though becoming much worse, are inadequately dealt with by medical services. Moreover, recent high demands for cultural and recreational activities since the South Korean government began enforcing a 5-day work week in 2004 have not been met, and this has caused additional employee stress (Choi, 2004).

Employees' psychosocial problems in terms of work, family, culture, and health are therefore likely to cause stress and eventually give rise to negative effects on their families and themselves. This stress tends to have a ripple effect, spreading to their work performance, resulting in absenteeism, worker turnover, low job commitment, a declining sense of responsibility, and industrial accidents (Moen, 1989).

Self-Esteem

There is no universally accepted conception of self-esteem, but many scholars define it as a self-evaluating attitude toward one's own value or importance (Coopersmith, 1967; Damon & Hart, 1982). The relation of self-esteem to stress and maladjustment is explained by Kaplan, Robbins, and Martin (1983) in two steps: firstly, stress decreases self-esteem, and reduced self-esteem consequently increases maladjustment. Stress also lessens self-esteem directly by impairing the social network that could provide one with support. That is, experiencing stress directly results in self-devaluation and in a deterioration of self-esteem and one's social network or adjustment, and finally in lowered self-esteem.

Organizational Commitment

Organizational commitment comprises a sense of conformity, attachment, affection, involvement, loyalty, identification, and affiliation. Buchanan (1974) defined *organizational commitment* as a strong emotional affection to the goals and values it pursues, to the role it performs, and to the organization itself, and it manifests itself as a psychological bond between a single member and an organization. Bateman and Strasser (1984) delineated it as loyalty to an organization, enthusiastic devotion to it, conformity to its goals and values, and the desire to remain its member. Levels of organizational commitment may therefore vary according to the degree of willingness to devote oneself to one's organization, to believe and accept its goals and values, and to become or desire to belong to it as a member.

Most research has noted that the establishment of a working system based on full commitment must be a vital element in the success of organizations. At the same time, they also indicated that organizational commitment is negatively influenced by stress at work (Fukami & Larson, 1984; Parker & Decotiis, 1983). It is thus a crucial strategy for human resource management to promote less stressful environments at work.

METHOD

Sampling

This study selected a public enterprise that was engaged in the construction and operation of expressway network in South Korea, recording the assets of $39,532,836,000 and the revenues of $2,981,120,000 in total in 2006 (Korea Expressway Corporation, 2007). Due to the diverse occupational categories this study sought to focus on, that is, ones ranging from manufacturing to service jobs, or from entry-leveled to high-ranked managers, it was appropriate to select the company that included each characteristic in these categories and to analyze problems the employees encountered in various situations.

A preliminary questionnaire was constructed based on previous literatures and focused group interviews, and a pilot study was conducted in May 2006. Then a final questionnaire was developed after we carefully revised the outcomes of the pilot study. Of the employees at the target company in the Seoul metropolitan area, 1,000 workers were randomly chosen, and the main survey was conducted in June 2006. Of the 730 questionnaires returned, 715 valid questionnaires were applied for the final analysis.

The samples were predominantly male (93.8%), and approximately 83.1% of the total were married 83.1% were married. The Korean workforce in the entire manufacturing industry is correspondingly male oriented, and the great majority are also married (Ministry of Labor, 2003). About 78.3% were reported to be in their thirties and forties, and most of the respondents had completed secondary (25.5%) or baccalaureate (56.6%) education. In terms of job classification, 127 workers (17.8%) were office related, 267 (37.3%) were engineering related, and 321 (44.9%) were technical related. The sample consisted mostly of entry (34.6%) or midlevel managers (59.5%) who have been with their firms for an average of 14.6 years.

Operational Definition and Measurement

The independent variables in this study were the workers' psychosocial problems experienced in the workplace or family. Employees' psychosocial problems indicated various obstacles that they directly confront in the workplace or family system. In total, 39 questions in regard to nine problems in three categories were formed to acquire sufficient data to analyze workers' psychosocial problems. Table 1 illustrates the categories and questions in detail.

TABLE 1 Categories and Questions Applied in the Survey

Category	Problem	Details
Workplace	Working system	Maladjustment of organizational changes
		Interpersonal problems
		Inefficient time management
		Misunderstanding of corporate policy/regulations
		Lack of job training
		Burden of side works
		Maladjustment of positions
		Lack of leadership
	Retirement	Retirement-related problems
		Lack of vocational guidance after retirement
	Workplace violence	Physical violence
		Verbal violence
		Sexual harassment
Family life	Family relationship	Marital conflicts
		Family conflicts
		Single parents' problems
		Divorced couples' problems
	Dependent care	Dual income families' separation problems
		Preschool children's care
		Children's schooling problems
		Children's education problems
		Elder care problems
		Lack of legal information
	Crises	Sudden death/accident of friends and families
		Unemployment of families
		Industrial disasters
		Financial/credit-related problems
Health & cultural life	Culture & leisure	Lack of recreation
		Lack of volunteer activities
		Lack of vacation/travel information
		Lack of cultural activities
	Medical service	Inaccessible medical service
		Lack of outside service in connection with company
		Rehabilitation problem
	Health	Mental health problems
		Alcohol problems
		Smoking problems
		Health care/fitness problems
		Dietary problems

The dependent variables for this study were workers' organizational commitment and self-esteem. To measure the degree of organizational commitment, this study applied the Organizational Commitment Questionnaire (OCQ) developed by Mowday, Steers, and Porter (1979). The Self-Esteem Scale (SES) developed by Rosenberg (1965) was used as well to estimate degrees of self-esteem.

To measure workers' stress, the mediator of this study, the Perceived Stress Scale (PSS), was applied. Developed by Cohen, Kamarck, and Mermelstein (1983), it has been widely used as the predicting factor for depression, social anxiety, and other related illnesses in various cultures. Finally, SPSS/ PC$^+$ 12.0 and Amos 5.0 were used for the analysis.

RESULTS

Model Test

To assess the convergent validity of each factor, the exploratory factor analysis (EFA) with the varimax rotation was applied. As presented in Table 2, internal consistency was tested as well by the reliability test, which that was required to confirm validity.

The maximum likelihood estimation, a coefficient calculation method in the structural equation model, was applied to assess the expediency of the proposed model. The result of the overall model test indicated that the proposed model was insufficient to be used as a reasonably fit model ($x^2 = 1960.89$, Goodness-of-Fit Index [GFI] = .833, Adjusted Goodness-of-Fit Index [AGFI] = .804, Normed Fit Index [NFI] = .758, Tucker-Lewis Index [TLI] = .771, Root Mean Square Error of Approximation [RMSEA] = .081). Consequently, we computed the Modification Index (MI) to obtain a more appropriate overall model, assuming that the measurement errors of available measurement

TABLE 2 Results of the Factor Analysis and Reliability Test

Factor		No. of items	Cronbach's α
Workplace	Work organization	8	.876
	Retirement problems	2	.851
	Workplace violence	3	.804
Family	Family relationships	3	.643
	Family care	6	.741
	Crisis problems	3	.858
Culture/health	Culture/leisure	4	.858
	Medical problems	3	.805
	Health problems	5	.858
Stress		6	.754
Organizational commitment		7	.881
Self-esteem		6	.812
Social support		19	.898

variables had correlations. Moreover, new paths between workers' self-esteem and organizational commitment, and between culture/health problems and work problems were found and linked to each other.

After a retesting of the overall model, we acquired a better fit than previous model $x^2 = 824.704$, GFI = .924, AGFI = .904, NFI = .898, TLI = .924, .924, RMSEA = .047). Also, after the chi-square difference test, it was found to have a difference value of 1,136.19, which significantly decreased, $df(23, 0.05) = 35.17$. Ultimately, this revised model was chosen as the most suitable. Table 3 shows the comparative results that the Fit Index generated between the original model and the revised model.

Testing the Measurement Model

The measurement model was tested by a confirmatory factor analysis (CFA) of the measurement variables of the set model. The standardized regression coefficient β values indicate how accurately the measurement instruments represented theoretical concepts. The values of the squared multiple correlator (SMC), a conceptual tool similar to communality in factor analysis, represented that the theory variable explained the measurement concept.

The results of the measurement model showed that the β values for each subcategory measuring workplace problems, family problems, culture/ health problems, stress, organizational commitment, and self-esteem were found to be statistically significant in the level of .001. This finding indicated that the measurement model was in fact appropriate for determining the theory variables.

Testing the Theory Model: The Original Structural Model

Summaries of the results of the hypotheses were shown in Table 4. First, Hypothesis 1, that is, the relation between workers' workplace problems and stress, was supported because the path coefficient was found to be significant ($t > 1.96$, $p < 0.05$), predicting that many problems in the workplace had significant effects on the increase of stress. Also, Hypothesis 2, regarding workers' family problems, and Hypothesis 3, regarding cultural and health problems, were found to have positive effects on stress. These findings were generally consistent with those in prior research (Carlson et al., 2000; Choi,

TABLE 3 Results of Fit Tests

Fit Index	χ^2	df	p	Q	GFI	AGFI	RMSEA	NFI	TLI
Original model	1960.89	345	.000	5.684	.833	.804	.081	.758	.771
Revised model	824.70	322	.000	2.561	.924	.904	.047	.898	.924

GFI = Goodness-of-Fit Index, AGFI = Adjusted Goodness-of-Fit Index, RMSEA = Root Mean Square Error of Approximation, NFI = Normed Fit Index, TLI = Tucker-Lewis Index.

TABLE 4 Summary of Hypotheses and Findings

Hypothesis	Path	Path Coefficient	Standard Errors	t Value
Hypothesis 1	Workplace problems →Stress	.276	.042	6.553***
Hypothesis 2	Family problems → Stress	.179	.064	2.820**
Hypothesis 3	Culture/health problems → Stress	.428	.111	3.861***
Hypothesis 4	Stress → Organizational commitment	−.127	.048	−3.009*
Hypothesis 5	Stress → Self-esteem	−.103	.028	−2.027**

*$p < .05$, **$p < .01$, ***$p < .001$.

2004; Myers, 1984; Paik & Choi, 2006; Voydanoff, 1989) and lead to the conclusion that workers' psychosocial problems are significant stress-producing factors.

Moreover, Hypotheses 4 and 5 predicted that stress would have significantly negative effects on both organizational commitment and self-esteem. The findings indicate that increased stress levels impeded the degree of workers' organizational commitment and damaged their self-esteem, finding which were consistent with the prior research (Burt, Cohen, & Bjorck, 1988; Parker & Decotiis, 1983; Roosa, Sander, Beals, & Short, 1988).

Additionally, self-esteem was found to have a positive effect on organizational commitment (path coefficient $= −0.401$, SE $= .047$, $t = 8.532$). As noted earlier in Murrell, Meeks, and Walker (1991), a high degree of self-esteem as an alternative resource alleviated negative behavior or promoted positive outcomes, while simultaneously representing the given individuals' level of mental health in itself.

Lastly, family problems had significantly negative effects on culture and health problems (path coefficient $= .313$, SE $= .072$, $t = 4.367$). This finding indicated that family problems were significant factors of negative effects on workers' cultural and health lives. Figure 1 following here shows a

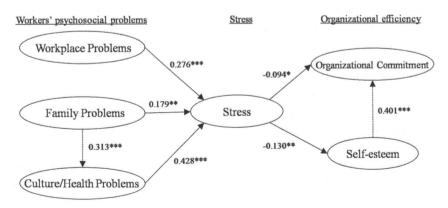

FIGURE 1 The revised model. *Note.* The elements marked by dotted lines are not statistically significant. *$p < .05$, **$p < .01$, ***$p < .001$.

summary of the test results of the hypotheses. The elements marked by dotted lines were used in the revised model.

SUMMARY

This study aimed to examine the psychosocial problems that workers encounter and to demonstrate how these problems affect stress, organizational commitment, and self-esteem.

Firstly, to achieve our goals, we derived a total of 39 questions from previous studies in relation to workers' psychosocial problems and from depth interviews with on-site workers. Then, using the EFA, we summarized these questions into 37 detailed subordinate questions and nine questions that the respondents responded to, and again categorized them into three sets; workplace problems, family problems, and health and cultural problems.

Secondly, problems that the workers have confronted were proven to influence stress. Of the various problems cited, workplace problems, such as the working system, retirement, and workplace violence problems turned out to be a serious stressor. Indeed, job insecurity in South Korea has been widespread because the early retirements and massive layoffs that occurred after the financial crisis in 1997.

Additionally, cultural and recreation problems, medical problems, and health problems were shown to affect the stress the workers experienced. This result indicated that the leisure-related programs that have been highlighted since the introduction of the five-day work week were also important in terms of workers' stress management, as were health and medical programs in the workplace.

Along with those problems, these results indicated that family issues, such as family relationships, child care, and unemployment, were as well main factors contributing to the workers' stress. These results showed that an employee's family problems were likely to have ramifications beyond the family boundary that extend to one's job activities. So far, South Korean workers' family problems have been viewed as the responsibility of each individual worker. In the future, however, workers' appropriate preventions and interventions to allay their family problems need to be applied to improve their productivity.

Third, this study confirmed that workers' psychosocial problems have had negative effects on both organizational commitment, a decisive factor in terms of organizational achievement and development, and on self-esteem, a dominating influence on individuals' motives and on the quality of life. Workers' stress that may be affected by problems that they encountered was proved to deteriorate their level of organizational commitment, as well as to damage their self-esteem. Considering the important roles self-esteem plays in the individual worker's successful job practice, appropriate intervention and management of their psychosocial problems should be practiced.

Lastly, given that this study notwithstanding focused on the effect of workers' psychosocial problems on stress, organizational commitment, and self-esteem, its covering of the various issues that workers confront in their workplaces was insufficient to permit an analysis with definitive results. Moreover, this study has another limitation in its counting of general demo-social factors, even though its data analysis through the structural equation model provided the advantage of acquiring power valid to explain covariations. Following studies should therefore overcome such limitations through a vast range of sampling and a thorough scrutiny of data on various applicable issues.

To sum up, employees have been suffering from serious levels of stress in their workplace, family, and leisure environments. These stresses brought deterioration in their degree of organizational commitment and a decrease in their self-esteem. Interventions in the psychosocial problems of workers and in their mental health should consequently no longer be delayed in order to both protect potential clients and promote company productivity.

In many economically advanced countries, EAPs were developed to deal with workers' psychosocial problems and to actively manage their stress on a corporate welfare level. EAPs have in fact played important roles in terms of organizational levels in securing and maintaining work forces, improving productivity, advancing labor-management relations, enhancing companies' images, and completing social responsibility in society (Googins & Godfrey, 1987; Saunders, Driskell, Johnston, & Salas, 1996; Van Den Bergh, 1995).

Because EAPs have proved their effectiveness in intervening in workers' psychosocial problems, the suggestions this study makes can provide meaningful alternatives for dealing with stress-related issues in workplaces in South Korea. However, such programs would have to be implemented differently from those initiated in Western examples since considerable differences in work environments and in particular in the problems workers confront do exist between Western societies and South Korea. Prior to the adoption of Western's EAPs, Korean companies should practice traditional EAP services like mental health improvement programs for workers and job stress management programs, and then continually strive to reach effective means of dealing with stress-related issues.

REFERENCES

Bateman, T., & Strasser, S. (1984). A longitudinal analysis of the antecedents of organizational commitment. *Academy of Management Journal, 27*(1), 95–112.
Buchanan, B. (1974). Building organizational commitment: The socialization of managers in work organization. *Administrative Science Quarterly, 19*(4), 533–546.

Burke, P. J. (1991). Identity process and social stress. *American Sociological Review*, 56(6), 836–849.

Burt, C. E., Cohen, L. H., & Bjorck, J. P. (1988). Perceived family environment as a moderator of young adolescents' life stress adjustment. *American Journal of Community Psychology*, 16(1), 101–122.

Carlson, D. S., Kacmar, K. M., & Williams, L. J. (2000). Construction and initial validation of a multidimensional measure of work-family conflict. *Journal of Vocational Behavior*, 56(2), 249–276.

Chang, S. J. (2002, May). *The present situation and condition of job stress among Korean employees*. Paper presented at Mental Health in the Workplace, symposium conducted at the meeting of the Korean Society for Preventive Medicine, Seoul, Korea.

Choi, S. C. (2004). Social service needs assessment to promote employee assistance programs in the Korean workplace. *Journal of Korean Social Welfare Administration*, 6(1), 71–103.

Choi, S. C. (2006). Applying needs assessment skills in the implementation of EAP structures: An examination of how to promote the growth of underdeveloped EAPs in Korean corporations. *Journal of Workplace Behavioral Health*, 21(2), 45–58.

Cohen, S., Kamarck, T., & Mermelstein, R. (1983). A global measure of perceived stress. *Journal of Health and Social Behavior*, 24(4), 385–396.

Coopersmith, S. (1967). *The antecedents of self-esteem*. San Francisco, CA: W.H. Freeman & Company.

Damon, W., & Hart, D. (1982). The development of self-understanding from infancy through adolescence. *Child Development*, 53(4), 841–864.

Googins, B., & Godfrey, J. (1987). *Occupational social work*. Englewood Cliff, NJ; Prentice-Hall.

Fukami, C. V., & Larson, E. W. (1984). Commitment to company and union: Parallel models. *Journal of Applied Psychology*, 69(3), 367–371.

House, J. S. (1981). *Work stress and social support*. Reading, MA: Addison-Wesley.

Kaplan, H. B., Robbins, C., & Martin, S. S. (1983, September). Antecedents of psychological distress in young adults: Self-rejection, deprivation of social support, and life event. *Journal of Health and Social Behavior*, 24, 230–244.

Kelly, B., Holbrook, J., & Bragen, R. (2005). Ceridian's experience in the integration of EAP, Work-Life and Wellness Programs. *Journal of Workplace Behavioral Health*, 20(1/2), 183–201.

Korea Expressway Corporation. (2007). Non-consolidated financial statements for the year ended December 31, 2006 and independent auditors' report. Seoul, Korea: Deloitte.

Latack, J. C. (1984). Career transitions within organizations: An exploratory study of work, nonwork, and coping strategies. *Organizational Behavior and Human Performance*, 34(3), 296–322.

McCroskey, J., & Scharlach, A. (1993). Family and work: Trends and prospects for dependent care. In P. A. Kurzman & S. H. Akabas (Eds.), *Work and well-being*, (pp. 153–169). Washington, DC: National Association of Social Workers.

Ministry of Labor. (2003). *White paper on labor*. Seoul, South Korea: Ministry of Labor.

Moen, P. (1989). Working parents: Transformations in gender roles and public policies in Sweden. Madison, WI: University of Wisconsin Press.

Mowday, R. T., Steers, R. M., & Porter, L. W. (1979). The measurement of organizational commitment. *Journal of Vocational Behavior, 14*(2), 224–247.

Murrell, S. A., Meeks, S., & Walker, J. (1991). Protective functions of health and self-esteem against depression in older adults facing illness or bereavement. *Psychology and Aging, 6*(3), 352–360.

Myers, D. W. (1984). Establishing and building employee assistance programs. West Port, CT: Quorum.

Paik, J. A., & Choi, S. C. (2006). The effect of the work and family conflict on overall stress and job satisfaction among workers with commuter marriage. *Korean Journal of Industrial and Occupational Psychology, 19*(4), 617–639.

Parker, D. F., & Decotiis, T. A. (1983). Organizational determinants of job stress. *Organizational Behavior and Human Performance, 32*(2), 160–177.

Roosa, M. W., Sander, I. N., Beals, J., & Short, J. L. (1988). Risk status of adolescent children of problem-drinking parents. *American Journal of Community Psychology, 16*(2), 225–239.

Rosenberg, M. (1965). *Society and the adolescent self-image.* Princeton, NJ: Princeton University Press.

Saunders, T., Driskell, J. E., Johnston, J. H., & Salas, E. (1996). The effect of stress inoculation training on anxiety and performance. *Journal of Occupational Health Psychology, 1*(2), 170–186.

U.S. Department of Labor (1990). *What work: Workplace without drugs.* Washington, DC: Author.

Van Den Bergh, N. (1995). Employee Assistance Programs. In R. L. Edwards (Ed.), *Encyclopedia of social work* (pp. 842–849). Washington, DC: NASW.

Voydanoff, P. (1989). Work and family: A review and expanded conceptualization. In E. B. Goldsmith (Ed.), *Work and family: Theory, research, and application,* (pp. 1–22). Newbury Park, CA: Sage.

Response to the Challenge of Training International EAP Professionals: An Online Certificate Program

DALE A. MASI, PhD

Masi Research Consultants, Inc., Boston, Massachusetts, USA

KENT CARLSON, BA

*Commonwealth of Massachusetts and Masi Research Consultants, Inc.,
Boston, Massachusetts, USA*

For the past 30 years, the first author has been training Employee Assistance Program (EAP) professionals. As the director of the EAP specialization at the University of Maryland School of Social Work, she was frequently asked about EAP training opportunities domestically and internationally. To meet this need, the author developed an online certificate program with Catholic University in Washington, DC. Subsequent to this writing, the program has moved to the School of Social Work at the University of Maryland, Baltimore (USA). The program has been offered for three years and has enrolled students from more than 25 countries and the United States. Most of the students are indigenous to their country, whereas some are U.S. civilian employees living and working overseas. The reader will see a firsthand account of how EAPs operate around the world, as viewed by local EAP practitioners.

The second author is Technology Associate, Masi Research Consultants, Inc., and Program Coordinator, Massachusetts Department of Conservation and Recreation. He is a technology business analyst and consultant implementing effective solutions for people, systems, and processes. He has worked in the public sector and private industry.

INTRODUCTION

Education is essential for a profession (Masi, 2011). The factual foundation of the efficacy of Employee Assistance Programs (EAPs) comes through its knowledge areas. Unfortunately, the knowledge base that many practicing professionals in the EAP field possess is not the specific type of knowledge that would help accelerate EAPs from a field of practice to an actual profession. Most EAP professionals learn from working on the job, not through conceptual understanding of the field. Many EAP professionals have never taken an academic course in EAPs (Jacobson & Attridge, 2010; Masi & Tisone, 2010).

Since 1985, the first author has been training professionals in the field of EAPs (Masi, 2002). As a professor at the University of Maryland, School of Social Work, she developed the EAP Specialization Program for social work masters-level students. The program averaged 25 to 30 students each year and, besides coursework, required a 3-day per week internship at an EAP.

From the beginning of her tenure at Maryland, she recognized that there was a critical need for more training (Masi & Maiden, 1985). The dearth of pedagogy in the field was not limited to the United States. At the time, she was lecturing in many countries for the U.S. State Department and was frequently being called by professionals overseas asking where they could receive further EAP training in their country. Her inability to provide an answer to that question has led to the development of the online curriculum and certificate program (described herein).

In 1988, along with directing the MSW program, she coordinated (with the School of Business) the development of a joint MBA/MSW degree program at the University of Maryland. An outgrowth of that cooperation between the two schools led to the development of an annual one-week continuing education residential program for EAP professionals. Professors from the Business School lectured on topics such as EAP marketing and human resources. The program was successful in attracting students from many countries (and the United States). However, it was an expensive option for students, as they were responsible for tuition and their own travel expenses. Despite this, there was a full enrollment for 10 years, but it was not nearly capable of satisfying the demand for training.

In the year 2000, the author was chairing the EAP Quality Assurance Committee for the Substance Abuse and Mental Health Services Administration (SAMHSA) (Manderscheid, Masi, Watkins, Carroll, & Santiago-Fernandez, 2005). The continuing need for training led her to approach SAMHSA about the development of a video-teleconference educational EAP program. The two-day lectures focused on EAP training and service delivery and attracted participants from several countries. SAMHSA and the University of Maryland ran the video-conference program for 2 years. Unfortunately, they could not charge for this because SAMHSA is a U.S. federal agency. Funds were not available to pay faculty for their time or cover any other operating expenses.

Meanwhile, online education was beginning to emerge, and the author realized that this development provided a unique option to offer EAP training to a truly global group of students and professionals (Masi, 2006).

NATIONAL CATHOLIC SCHOOL OF SOCIAL SERVICE

A member of the Catholic University alumni office who had heard about the author's interest in an online program contacted her (an alumna of the school) and suggested that she meet with the dean and discuss the possibility of providing the program through the university's National Catholic School of Social Service (NCSSS). Founded in 1918, NCSSS is one of the oldest schools of social work in the United States. The dean of NCSSS was enthusiastic about the possibility, and the author (through her firm Masi Research Consultants) entered into a contractual agreement with the University for the delivery of an online certificate training program regarding EAPs. Masi Research (MASI) specializes in the design, evaluation, and teaching of EAPs.

Under the arrangement, the university and MASI have specific roles. NCSSS is responsible for providing access to Blackboard (the web-based platform upon which the courses are offered), handles student registration and payments, and attains the approvals for the awarding of continuing education units and professional development hours credit. MASI develops the curriculum, markets to its network, teaches the courses, and provides its own technical support for the delivery of the electronic material.

Recently, the National Association of Social Workers (NASW) has joined with NCSSS and MASI to publicize the program to its 150,000 members, through its EAPrefer Program. NASW is also sponsoring webinars to recruit social workers into the EAP field.

The venture is now beginning its fourth year. Most interestingly, in addition to students from the United States, the course has registered men and women from 26 different countries, a fulfillment of the goal to be offering training that is accessible around the world.

TECHNOLOGY/CURRICULUM

The certificate program includes two courses (4 weeks each): EAPs in the New Millennium and EAP Optional Services. The first course covers the essential ingredients and core technology of EAPs. The second covers optional services that EAPs may offer, such as work/life and online counseling. The content for each course was developed by MASI, and each has a syllabus, journal articles, handouts, and discussion topics. Each week, a PowerPoint lecture of approximately 35 slides (with extensive notes) is presented to the class. Students are expected to read the current lecture and the recommended articles related to the lecture content, and participate in one or more discussion board forums.

The program is conducted on Blackboard. Using common applications like Microsoft Office and Adobe Acrobat to develop course material has meant few (if any) additional applications or plug-ins are needed beyond one of the prominent internet browsers. Syllabi and lectures were prepared in Microsoft Word or PowerPoint. Course introduction videos were prepared with the Panopto video capture software. References to journals, articles, other readings, and research are cited with hyperlinks or scanned and saved as Acrobat PDF files. As a result, at the end of the program, each student has an "EAP library." The program features one written assignment, described later in this article.

Following registration, a unique online account is created for each student. Documents are uploaded to the modified classroom shell and instructions guide students to current material. Settings can be used to automatically reveal course material on a specific date. Week 1 material is revealed on the first day of class, week 2 on the eighth day, and so on. Students can access the material on their own schedule, as the class is asynchronous. Discussion board forum topics are seeded with a starter thread. This initial thread starts the discussion much like a live question from the professor to a class full of students. Students comment and reply to each other, and each student comment is responded to by the faculty member. The discussion boards in each of the courses have been extremely lively. This is the most critical part of online learning: the interaction between the students in this forum really makes the learning "come alive" for them, build associations with one another, learn each other's backgrounds, and create a community.

Student technical support problems related to the use of the university's Blackboard website have been minimal. Of note, the difference between the frequency and type of technical difficulties accessing or using the Blackboard website by students inside or outside the United States is negligible.

THE STUDENTS

Countries Represented

China had the most number of students (six), all from Hong Kong. Other countries had several enrollees, such as Indonesia, Trinidad, Germany, and Greece.

The first two students to register were from Slovenia. Interestingly, an early registrant was an active-duty U.S. Navy serviceman serving as chief of mental health services on an aircraft carrier in international waters with 3,000 men and women on board. At certain times during the course the Navy would shut down the Internet, and he would be out of touch, but always returned and contributed a great deal.

From the very first class, there was a variety of countries and continents that were represented, which stimulated the discussions. Many of the students commented how pleased they were to see so many other countries represented in the class.

Over three years, in addition to numbers of U.S. registrants, international students from the following countries have enrolled:

- Argentina
- Azerbaijan
- Bahamas
- Barbados
- Bermuda
- Canada
- China (Hong Kong)
- France
- Germany
- Greece
- Indonesia
- Italy
- Kazakhstan
- Mongolia
- New Zealand
- Japan (Okinawa)
- The Philippines
- Portugal
- Russia
- Senegal
- Slovenia
- South Korea
- St. Lucia
- Trinidad/Tobago
- U.S. Aircraft Carrier in International Waters

Students' Educational Background

Regardless of country of origin, the educational level of the students was impressive. All of the students had a minimum of a bachelor's degree, and most had done master's work or higher (though there was no minimum-educational requirement for the program). Even with such credentials as the following, they still thought it necessary to enroll in classes on EAPs.

- doctors of philosophy: public health and social work
- doctor of education in counselor education
- doctor of medicine: psychiatrist

- masters of social work
- masters of arts in clinical/counseling/educational psychology
- master of business administration
- masters of science in human resources and occupational psychology
- bachelor of arts

Students' Positions

It was encouraging to discover so many international professionals who wanted to expand their knowledge of EAP service delivery and history, even though many were already working in the field. The following list illustrates the breadth of the students' careers.

18 EAP workers
4 U.S. military contractors
Lecturer in social work
U.S. Navy
Police officer in Royal Police Force
Educational researcher
Project worker in developing country
Psychiatrist, private practice
Professor on sabbatical from university
Freelance consultant in human capital management
Psychotherapist running a psych-support program in pediatric oncology
Counseling psychologist at a nongovernmental organization working with
    victims of human trafficking, family violence, incest, and sexual abuse.

DISCUSSION THREADS

Each course has generated approximately 500 student comments and faculty responses.[1] A sample of these Discussion Board questions and student comments follow:

Discussion Question: Ethics: Do You Think the EAP Field Today Has Any Ethical Issues? (Employee Assistance Professionals Association [EAPA], 2009; Ethics monograph, 1996; Sharar, White, & Funk, 2002)

Slovenia[2]: I have a basic ethical question. In capitalism, where by default we
    have two antagonistic sides—owners (managers/supervisors) and work-
    ers, is it really possible to work equally for both sides, when one side is
    paying for your work but the other side is obviously weaker?
Germany: It is so important to have an ethical framework! The companies often
    put pressure on the EAP because they want information (not on individuals,

but they want detailed reports to see what is happening in their company). It is sometimes difficult to convince them that we cannot give them that much detail. Also we are confronted with the question of telling the company how much it is saving because the EAP was used. This sometimes brings up ethical issues, because one doesn't really want to discuss things like: How much is the value of an employee that did not commit suicide because he had access to counseling at the moment when he needed it most?

Greece: In Greece, there are some mental health professionals that are practicing without having licensure or even sufficient training in the area that they claim as a specialization. In addition, we sometimes face some ethical issues regarding our multiple roles: we serve managers and employees as well as EAP providers.

Slovenia: Ethical issues can occur when EAP staff is trying to save some money and is therefore signing contracts with cheaper subcontractors that may not be the most appropriate and competent. Consequently people are not getting quality service. Ethical issues can also arise if an EAP counselor doesn't have proper knowledge and training, for example, about alcohol or drug abuse and, despite that, is counseling people with those kinds of problems.

New Zealand: Balancing the needs of the employer and the employee through the work done by a clinician (counselor/psychologist) is potentially an ethical dilemma. The challenge is often about confidentiality and how to manage and balance how much remains confidential especially around issues of power and who holds it. There are cases where an employee's behavior is perceived to be (and often is) unacceptable in the workplace. I have seen aggressive employees attempt to hold their roles through intimidation and threat. Equally I have heard some managers put challenging behaviors and demands on their employees. Who is right and how are these issues best resolved?

Greece: I absolutely agree with the vital importance of the client filling out the Statement of Understanding, the Release of Information, and Consent Form at the beginning of the first session. The client/employee and the organization must know the rights of the EAP counselor to disclose information under certain circumstances. As one of the articles mentions, it is unfortunately very difficult to control the affiliate EAP counselor: some of them are not always familiar with the procedures and the forms to be given to the served employee.

Regarding anonymity, take as an example a factory's onsite counseling: it has been observed by some EAP affiliates that sometimes employees find it hard to approach this EAP service and hesitant to visit because they must first go to their supervisors to ask for permission and then go to the HR manager or director to sign the permission, which is like taking a short sick-leave/ time-off from work to visit the EAP counselor.

Hong Kong: Exemption to confidentiality issues: We have a mechanism that is a crisis response team to discuss whether there are justified reasons to breach the confidentiality clause under the following conditions: (a) People with high/imminent suicidal risk, (b) people who pose harm to the public/others and (c) document/records requested by the court. I think it is crucial always to have collective/organizational responsibilities on these important issues.

Argentina: One of our concerns is related to EAP's legal responsibility in cases of suicidal risk. Let's assume the EAP assesses telephonically only, refers the client to an emergency service (psychiatric) external resource, and makes sure that a family member is informed: What is EAP's legal responsibility if the client harms himself or commits suicide? What if the family member ignores the warning? Is EAP's responsibility the same as if the client has had face-to-face sessions or is it reduced because of the telephonic assessment and referral? As EAP is not a known service in Argentina, there are no laws that regulate our practice yet. How does this work in other countries?

France: Because of the strong responsibilities of EAP providers who are partly in charge of employees' health, there certainly are ethical and legal issues in the EAP field. In France for instance, employers have a "duty" statement (performance obligation) regarding their employees' health. For example, if an employee commits suicide for professional reasons, the CEO could be sentenced to imprisonment. Obviously, in spite of the duty statement, the court will be much more accommodating with an employer that has a strong EAP than a company that does not.

Hong Kong: What should be done in response to a request from a Human Resource manager seeking consultation on what HR can do to determine if the company needs to report the case to police after terminating a staff member discovered to have several thefts in the company?

Slovenia: I would like to comment on the problem with these "anticapitalistic" system values, as we have bumped into this once at our supervision meeting. In our small team of counselors most of the counselors are younger and from the "new generation" (Slovenia was a socialistic country and has been capitalistic only since the nineties); the older counselors gained most of their work experience (and lived most of their lives) in the socialistic society. Discussing the counseling strategies for cases with problems such as work overload or life/work issues, the two groups of counselors took quite different positions. The older counselors were much more sympathetic to the worker.

Discussion Question: Core Technology: Do You Think This Is an Appropriate Conceptual Basis for the EAP Field? Include Your Comments about the Optional Services Listed in the Lecture (Roman & Blum 1988)

Slovenia: I agree that the Core Technology is an appropriate conceptual basis. I especially agree with training and assistance to the work organization's leadership and the use of constructive confrontation. In Slovenia, Wellness is for the privileged—it is not covered by insurance and you have to pay for it, except for physiotherapy after accidents. So I think it would be a great progress if we could include Wellness into EAP programs in Slovenia.

Germany: I like the Core Technology and think it is important for the EAP profession. I understood from my colleague that they are not very popular in Europe in the EAP community. I don't understand where the resistance comes.

Portugal: In Portugal I work as an external EAP provider and we are trying to educate the market about the value of EAPs. I work mainly with private companies that are beginning to accept that these programs are very helpful with problems, but they only accept it when they have "tried everything else." In our field the EAP Core Technology is adopted with care, as the market is not mature. Having an EAP is viewed as a threat because it is seen as a failure of the company to take care of its employees. Even when I explain the impact in well-being, productivity, performance or return on investment the skepticism is enormous. Promoting EAPs is an amazing and great challenge.

US Aircraft Carrier: The military's adaptation of constructive confrontation (intrusive leadership) will not work in the private sector. In the military there is a greater sense of ownership of our employees . . . . I believe the best EAP counselors will be highly visible people in an organization with a genuine talent for reaching employees through the use of the Core Technology. EAP counselors will be caring people who are not afraid to get involved–constructive confrontation–and diffuse issues before they overwhelm the employee.

Following my review of the lecture and reading assignments I believe the Core Technology of EAP is on solid footing. While I have not been for-mally trained as an EAP counselor, I will say that I see many parallels with the Core Technology in my current capacity as a senior enlisted Sailor in the US Navy. As Roman and Blum suggest, follow-up and supervisor involvement are key contributors to turning poor performance around and salvaging a good worker.

Hong Kong: The Core Technology is not popular in Hong Kong, and even less so in mainland China, as employees' benefits are sometimes perceived as a liability instead of capital in the commercial balance sheet. Employers are willing to pay more for rent but not for services. Deploying an EAP system and technology in the commercial, edu-cational, and government industries is definitely not a priority (in Hong Kong).

Slovenia: Those who are involved in the EAP field should recognize the importance of Core Technology in the EAP profession no matter who developed it. In my opinion such prejudices from some European

EAPs are quite immature and foolish. Not all of us from Europe are so narrow-minded.

New Zealand: I too think that trauma (critical incident stress management) needs to be a core technology for EAPs. We have had quite an increase in critical incident calls over the last two years. This is in addition to the earthquake that happened in one of our major cities, Christchurch.

However, we take a much less interventionist role with our client organizations. Commoditization of EAPs is high and we no longer offer "consultation with, training of, and assistance to work organization leaders." It is no longer a Core Technology for an EAP here in New Zealand. Approximately 90% of the counselling work that comes through our national free phone is self-referral. It is rare for our EAP to provide an intervention directly to management in our client organizations for this type of referral - unless we need to break our confidentiality agreement (at risk to self or others). The place where an EAP is best able to influence individual managers/HR and supervisors are through the 10% of referrals that are formally managed for specific expert consultation.

Greece: What Roman & Blum introduced is a good first attempt to describe the conceptual basis for the EAP field. The core EAP services include the basic components of the presence and implementation of an EAP in a work organization.

Commenting on the optional services, I would say that many EAP services are mentioned and some of them could be set under the same umbrella. For example: Welfare-to-Work programs could be along with the Wellness programs and Work/Life programs, since all these services together promote wellness, work-life balance and well-being strategies; the drug free workplace and SAP services might be considered together; conflict management/violence prevention may be connected with the risk management, because violence in the workplace, bullying, conflicts, impaired relationships between employees and many other issues are considered as risks for an organization. Could they all together be under a wider category of psychosocial & behavioral risk assessment/management service?

Furthermore, I suggest coaching as another service to be offered for executives and managers, and expatriate support services for managers and their families (local and abroad).

As for the outplacement service, I think it is appropriately in our list, since this kind of service is extremely useful for our clients especially during hard times of downsizing and early retirements.

Hong Kong: EAPs originated from the occupational social work field where the concepts of "welfare," advocacy for justice," and "equality" should offer some guiding, underlying principles in promoting the wellbeing of employees. I am curious to know how the field has evolved and come up with an agreement that "productivity" and "work performance" became the highlight of the field. As you may know, there often is conflict between the employer and the employee. As an EAP professional, I am always wondering about the values for which we should stand.

I think that management consultation service is of growing importance in the field and it is a powerful tool to mitigating supervisor-subordinate tension and counseling them to a common solution to benefit both.

Concerning the Core Technology of EAPs, I would like to add crisis-care service as well. Service for expatriates and pre-retirement programs could also be included in view of the globalization trend in the world.

Argentina: Roman and Blum write that "the Core Technology identifies those unique functions of EAPs that differentiate them from other human resource activities in the workplace." In Argentina as in other countries of Latin America, providing clients with a clear explanation of EAP Core Technology is fundamental, as EAPs have developed a very short time ago here and boundaries are still unknown. Argentina has a very long and strong history of psychotherapy, mostly psychoanalytic models, and this makes it even more difficult to differentiate EAP services from clinical practice. One of our challenges is educating organizations about the Core Technology of EAPs.

Another peculiarity of Latin American countries is about trends in utilization. Over the years we have observed a pattern of receiving more legal consults than psychological and financial, and this is the same for very different kind of companies. The average pattern is 62% legal consults, 23% psychological consults, 8% financial consults and the rest are informative consults. For this reason, we believe that in our culture legal counseling should be considered part of the Core Technology.

I agree with other participants that critical incidents stress debriefing should be included in the Core Technology.

Philippines: I am also not sure where to draw the line between "short term intervention" and psychological counseling. What is covered in "short term intervention" in the first place? In the Philippines, very few people go to counseling on their own account, and if they do, they do not have many sessions. They are not willing to pay for it. So they might as well get their therapy through the EAP. It's the most helpful thing we can do for people.

In addition, as I mentioned in a comment to another thread, screening employees for emotional fitness before being assigned abroad, and preparing employees to be assigned abroad, are valuable EAP services. For those non-accompanying family members, the EAP can be a beneficial support. If the destination country has no EAP, then we may offer online counseling to the expatriated employee.

Senegal: I believe Core Technology is an appropriate basis for EAP, for upfront Roman and Blum illustrate the fact that EAPs must offer a broad and open view to employee care. The Core Technology functions are interested in the organization as a whole and take into account the employees, the supervisors, and the system. This allows the EAP specialist to understand and offer more appropriate assistance to the employee. In contrast, some more traditional systems automatically stigmatize the employee and ask "What is dysfunctional with the employee?" rather than "What in the system is making the employee unproductive?"

In the lecture, the graph represents several optional services. However, I would dissociate/remove any service that could be offered by the local social services. My concern is that employees not rely only on services provided through the EAP. Employees should be encouraged to be as autonomous as possible and they should learn to have a medical and social back-up independent of the workplace in order to avoid putting themselves in a precarious situation if they were to ever lose their job position.

Russia: I believe the Core Technology provides a solid base for EAP services. This especially applies to new companies in need of guidance. Personally, I can say that living in a rather chaotic environment here, it has done wonders to reduce my anxiety to have solid standards to match and keep the company moving along.

Optional services, I believe, can vary. There are certain ones that benefit any company, such as stress management or wellness. Then there are those that are needed more in certain cultures or companies—for example, our substance abuse program is usually used by large plants and factories that are based in small towns where people unfortunately feel that they have nothing else to do, and there are higher safety concerns. Our expat-support program is most needed in the city, for managerial staff who have been sent from other countries and have trouble adjusting (Russia is definitely not expat friendly).

Trinidad/Tobago: Based on my EAP experience on the island of Tobago, EAP Core Technology is definitely crucial especially as it relates to confidentiality of employees/client personal issues. The island of Tobago is very small and consists of a population where everyone either knows you or is related to you ... therefore EAP Services would not be successful if clients felt their personal problems could not be addressed under extremely confidential conditions ... which also includes the location of the EAP office. Therefore once EAP clients are reassured of confidentiality it is easier to address and treat their personal issues thereby improving work performance, employee/employer relations and by extension the work environment.

Japan: The Core Technology functions are effective for the EAP field. As the assessment function is imperative to good treatment planning and outcome; a solid foundation or canon from which to function is imperative to establish expectations and gauge effectiveness. Additionally, it sets a standard for the professional and those that engage in and with the activities of EAPs.

Barbados: The Core Technology is the raison d'etre for EAPs and designed to help restore employees to optimal functioning in the workplace. Hence it is an effective base for the EAP field. It does indeed set EAP apart from other human resource activities in the workplace and this is essential in helping EAP maintain its professional identity.

I like it that one of the EAP functions includes "consultation with, training of, and assistance to work organizations' leadership (managers and supervisors, and union stewards)" who are part of the environment of the troubled employee and who should all seek to improve employee functioning and well-being.

South Korea: Core Technology is mostly what I find to be the day-to-day things of an EAP. As for other functions I find they change day-to-day. I find working overseas I assist a lot of clients with just finding the resources within the community that they cannot get on post. The key is to find resources that can assist in English or have available translation services. Korea has a great off-post health care system and many of the hospitals have international clinics to assist.

As for optional services such as drug testing, I do not think an EAP should be part of the drug testing process: the EAP needs to be a neutral party in the process in case a person tests positive, so that the EAP could be involved to assist the client with what happens next in the process.

Discussion Question: Comment on the Certified Employee Assistance Professional (CEAP) Process. Is It Something of Value in Your Country?

Slovenia: I think that the CEAP process is necessary and if we can succeed as an independent EAP provider I am sure that we will have the same process of certification.

Germany: The CEAP process is not relevant in our country. I have heard of two counselors/EAP managers in Germany that ran through the process. They did not renew, because it is a lot of work and nobody cares in Germany. I also heard that the language barrier is very high (not easy for a non-native speaker to pass the test) and that it focuses a lot on American legislation. The German market is in a process now where the EAP providers have to differentiate, so that the customer can choose the model that fits him best. The CEAP process would not be helpful in this stage, because it would suggest to the customer that the CEAP is relevant in Germany while this has not been discussed yet ... we would just take something from America and assume that it fits here, which it does not necessarily do.... My team leader says that there has never been any discussion about the CEAP in the Employee Assistance European Forum (EAEF).

Greece: CEAP process is the official credential that represents the EA profession and demonstrates ability and mastery of the body of knowledge required for competence in EAP practice. A certain level of commitment is really necessary to understand the EAP model.

Greece: I agree with the point that CEAP is essential for protecting the EA professional from people who do not know the EA field, its philosophy, the services, the real aims and missions, and also protecting the client, employee and families. . . . I wonder why internships do not count towards EAP experience in the CEAP certification. . . . In Greece, client organizations do not ask for CEAP certification.

Hong Kong: Having the CEAP does not only demonstrate that the EA professionals possess the kind of professional skills needed to offer appropriate and confidential assessment, clinical intervention, referral and case management services, but that they also subscribe to the CEAP code of conduct and are accountable for our ethical behavior.

Argentina: The CEAP is fundamental for EAP professionals. Certification always improves quality of services and makes sure the professionals are doing what they are supposed to do. David Sharar's writings show clearly that the knowledge of many affiliates regarding EAP theory and practice is weak. Only 18% of the affiliates asked said that they were "very familiar" with EAP core technology, 37% are "not familiar at all," and 26% were "a little familiar." I am sure that in Argentina and the rest of Latin America, the percentage of respondents saying "not familiar at all" would be even higher. I hope CEAP spreads to all countries as soon as possible.

Philippines: Yes, I think the CEAP is very valuable, to professionalize what we do. I would say EAP is only starting in the Philippines and it is good to start right.

Hong Kong: Yes, the CEAP process is of value in Hong Kong. This is relatively new to us though it has been introduced in the 1980s. I hope the participation in CEAP helps to enhance the professional standard of the EAP services . . . having said that, the requirement for CEAP is really hard and challenging for me.

Discussion Question: Accreditation: What Do You Think Can Be Done to Convince the EAP Field that Accreditation Is the Responsible Professional Approach? (Council on Accreditation, 2014)

Slovenia: I think that the importance of accreditation is well-known. A contemporary problem is that pricing is more important than the quality. I see the solution in legislation.

Slovenia: For now there is only one company offering EAP services in Slovenia. I think that soon some people will see an opportunity to earn money with providing EAP services. My biggest concern is that in no time there will appear numerous so-called EAPs without accreditation. Yes, maybe the best option to prevent this is legislation but we all know that unfortunately that takes time. By that time the damage is already done. Is there any other option to deal with that problem?

New Zealand: Accreditation is essential for an EAP to market itself as the fully professional organization it purports to be. EAPs work with the mental health of employees. Having a process that makes EAPs accountable is highly desirable. Businesses like well-run, credible providers, and I suspect that having an acknowledged accreditation would enhance an EAP's reputation. While commoditization of EAPs is the norm, that is no reason to not pursue accreditation.

Accreditation will ensure quality clinicians, minimize complaints, enable internal systems to be monitored effectively, help managers find and manage poor processes and procedures, provide incentives to develop different or more effective systems, and help integrate the organization as a whole.

Greece: I have never thought that I would have to justify this. From the beginning of my work in the EAP field I heard about Standards and Accreditation (S&A). I strongly believe that the only way to protect organizations from charlatans is the presence of strong professional associations, like EAPA and EAEF, the setting of S&A, and obliging private and public sectors to consider them before buying an EAP. In the EU, EAPs are still growing: this can be a blessing since we can prevent malpractice by promoting Buyer's Guides. Also, EU-OSHA and other large agencies related to health and safety legislatives should include EAPs in their directives and projects. There is no better argument for following accreditation standards than the threat of paying penalties if an EAP provider company does not follow the S&A of the profession.

Philippines: The Philippines is a long, long way from the time when accreditation will be a common practice. But it's something to look forward to!

Bermuda: The predominant attitude can sometimes seem to be "why do we need someone to tell us how to do what we do?" My response to that is simple.

In this day and age, so many people are claiming to provide services without actually being held accountable. For example, in Bermuda there are currently four programs stating that they provide EAP services. In my opinion, only one of these programs actually does so. We decided this year to pursue accreditation as a means of distinguishing ourselves from the other companies and proving that we meet the standards.

My job is currently in the accreditation process through the Council on Accreditation (COA), and it is hard work! I think often programs can become content with the work they do, and do not want/wish/see the need to push themselves further into accreditation.

STUDENT VISITS

As part of the coursework, each student was also required to submit a paper based on the student's visit to a local EAP (either an in-house or external program). Students were asked to meet with key staff people (preferably the director) and conduct an interview about the EAP's operation (including the EAP model in place, staffing, training, and evaluation methods). If there was not an EAP in the student's area, the student was to visit a human resource professional at a local company. Due to privacy and confidentiality issues, in summarizing the major observations from the visits by the international students, specific students will not be identified.

A number of students interviewed HR personnel, since EAPs were not accessible. Several of the EAPs that were interviewed ranged from those that had been in business since the 1980s (Elder Associates and Shepell•fgi). to others that were extremely new, in business for only one or 2 years. Several programs existed in U.S. multinational corporations that have actually been responsible for the development of international EAPs (Chevron is one example).

Many of the EA and HR professionals interviewed expressed concerns about employee confidentiality. Interestingly, many of the programs in place required that an employee get permission from the HR and/or the supervisor in order to utilize the EAP. In addition to confidentiality, the idea of a stigma associated with mental illness (and, by extension, use of the EAP) was also of concern.

There was strong support for accreditation. Several of the EAPs interviewed were already COA-accredited (Shepell•fgi, Elder Associates, and EAP Bermuda). Many of the programs had full-time staff, so the use of affiliates was not found to be the same problem in some EAPs as it is in the United States.

Recruiting staff is a problem in many Eastern European countries because the teaching of psychology is based on theory, and not on practice and internship, so many graduates have not met with an actual client. As pointed out before, the conflict between the socialistic versus capitalistic view came up often as a concern, especially for those EAPs that wanted to simply act as employee-advocates.

The programs in the Balkans believed they would see growth in EAPs because of the strong support they were receiving from the European Union.

CONCLUSION

Students continually raised important questions and introduced issues that the EAP field should consider. Several students commented on the inherent conflict between the socialistic versus capitalistic philosophy in an employee assistance program. Even in the United States, the author sometimes encounters this with students who want to defend workers (clients) over management, regardless of the issue.

Even though written in 1988, Roman and Blum's EAP Core Technology was perceived by most students as valuable. They frequently suggested that trauma response services should be included. One of the most thought-provoking comments was from the student who asked how the field evolved into one in which productivity and work performance were the highest goals, when it developed from occupational social work/alcoholism, where advocacy and concern for the welfare of the client was the main focus.

International students, and their U.S. counterparts, did not have a clear understanding of the difference between CEAP certification (meant for individuals) and accreditation (for programs). They supported both, often confusing them. They never faltered, however, in their belief of the need for oversight and monitoring of the individual EAP practitioner and the program itself.

Education has been sorely lacking for EAPs, and almost nonexistent in many areas of the world. There is no doubt that online learning is growing exponentially. The authors see the online program as described as one answer to meet this need. It has opened our eyes even more than ever of the need for EAP education. As the online program evolves, we intend to refine the technology and add more sophisticated tools to the program. We will also keep the cost at an amount that is affordable for all EAPs, regardless of the country of origin. We then can look forward to a universal understanding of EAPs and fostering an international conversation across country boundaries.

NOTES

1. To preserve anonymity student names are not used, and comments taken from the Open Discussion board are paraphrased.

2. More than one comment from the same country is due to multiple students from that country in the course, or the same student responding to another's thread.

REFERENCES

Council on Accreditation. (2014). *Eighth edition standards*. Retrieved from http://coanet.org/standard/eap

Employee Assistance Professionals Association (EAPA). (2009). *EAPA code of ethics*. Retrieved from http://www.eapassn.org/files/public/EAPACodeofEthics0809.pdf

Ethics monograph. (1996). Houston, TX: Houston Chapter of the Employee Assistance Professionals Association. Page 1.

Jacobson, J., & Attridge, M. (2010, August). Employee assistance programs (EAPs): An allied profession for work/life. In S. Sweet & J. Casey (Eds.), *Work and family encyclopedia*. Chestnut Hill, MA: Sloan Work and Family Research Network. Retrieved from http://wfnetwork.bc.edu/encyclopedia_entry.php?id= 17296&area=All

Manderscheid, R., Masi, D., Watkins, G., Carroll, C., & Santiago-Fernandez, E. (2005). The employee assistance industry alliance: Context, history, and initial vision. *Employee Assistance Quarterly, 19*(3), 1–10.

Masi, D. (2002, May/June). Professional education: The key to developing conceptual thinking. *EAP Association Exchange, 32*(3), 23–25.

Masi, D. (2006). New initiatives in the EAP field. *Behavioral Healthcare, 26*(4), 23–24.

Masi, D. (2011). Redefining the EAP field. *Journal of Workplace Behavioral Health, 26*(1), 1–9.

Masi, D., & Maiden, R. P. (1985, July/August). EAP specialization at the University of Maryland. *EAP Digest: The Voice of Employee Assistance Programs*, 63–64.

Masi, D. & Tisone, C. (Eds). (2010). *The 4th international employee assistance compendium*. Boston, MA: Masi Research Consultants, Inc.

Roman, P., & Blum, T. (1988). The core technology of employee assistance programs. *The ALMACAN, 19*(8), 17–22.

Sharar, D., White, W., & Funk, R. (2002). Business ethics and employee assistance: A national survey of issues and challenges. *Employee Assistance Quarterly, 18*(2), 39–59.

Group Characteristics and Mental Health of Chinese Expatriates in Africa and Central Asia: A Multisite, Multiyear Study

PEIZHONG LI, PhD

Chestnut Global Partners, China, Shanghai, China

DAVID A. SHARAR, PhD

Chestnut Global Partners, Bloomington, Illinois, USA

JIE ZHANG, MBA

Chestnut Global Partners, China, Beijing, China

This study examines the mental health status of Chinese expatriate workers stationed in Africa and Central Asia in relation to their demographic and occupational characteristics. Data were collected from expatriates working for two large Chinese companies in different locations over 5 years. Two studies provide a consistent profile of Chinese expatriates in terms of gender makeup, age distribution, family structure, education, and management positions. Study 1 shows that women, managers, and more educated expatriates report more symptoms of psychological distress than men, nonmanagers, and employees with less education. Study 2 examines more specific symptoms among managers and nonmanagers across different contexts, that is, when they are on duty, vacationing, and prior to deployment. Expatriates on duty fared worse than their vacationing or predeployment colleagues. This trend was more prominent among the managers. Implications of the findings with respect to improving the working and living conditions and mental health assistance for this group are discussed.

INTRODUCTION

Resource-rich and underdeveloped countries of Africa, South America, Central Asia, and the Middle East have seen rapid increases in Chinese investments and business activities, especially in the mining and construction sectors. This increase is partly fueled by China's need for oil, copper, gold, and other minerals as the country becomes a major manufacturing center in the world (Sun, 2014). Meanwhile, China has emerged as one of the largest providers of economic aid to many African countries (e.g., Brautigam, 2011). Chinese foreign aid often comes in the form of low-interest loans for building infrastructures in exchange for the rights to develop the recipient countries' mineral resources (Piao, 2006). Resource development and infrastructure building financed by China are mostly contracted to Chinese companies (Sun, 2014; Yi. 2011). Operations in these sectors require a large number of Chinese personnel to "work on the ground" in foreign- recipient countries. As a result, a growing number of Chinese workers and managers are stationed abroad for extended periods of time as part of their job assignment. Although the potential impact of Chinese investments and economic activities on the local communities in the recipient countries have become a subject of intense international debate in economic and political sectors (Brautigam, 2011; Sun, 2014), the impact on Chinese expatriates has received little public attention. This study takes the first step to fill this gap in our knowledge. Understanding Chinese expatriates' mental health and its contributing factors should help employers improve working conditions, safety, productivity, and the ultimate success of expatriate assignments. This information will also help clinicians provide more effective assistance and intervention to this population.

Compared with domestic-based employees, expatriates face unique personal and professional challenges. These may include work–life balance issues such as increased workload, separation from significant others, and also difficulties in adjusting to the natural, social, and cultural environments of the host country (Black & Gregersen, 1999; Black & Mendenhall, 1991). Research with U.S. samples shows that expatriates are at greater mental health risks than their domestic-based counterparts (Truman, Sharar, & Pompe, 2011). Adjustment may prove more challenging for Chinese expatriates because of their difficult working and living conditions, including uncomfortably hot or cold climates as well as a lack of basic services, amenities, and recreation opportunities. Most Chinese expatriates in the mining and construction sectors live in closed campuses near their worksites. Their movements outside the campuses are often restricted due to safety concerns, language barriers, and regulations from employers. Adding to their stress, most Chinese expatriates leave their families at home while working overseas, reuniting with families only during vacations. The long-distance travel and lack of regular physical family contact increase their stress. Political and military conflicts in some of the host countries constitute another source of worry and threats to safety. Some expatriates have been evacuated from host countries due to armed conflicts. A tiny fraction of them have been kidnapped and released only after ransoms were paid. News about these incidents feed an aura of hardship and danger among this expatriate group.

Despite compelling reasons for concern about the mental health status of Chinese expatriates, factors that potentially protect them from the negative impact of working overseas also exist. The expatriates have accepted their assignments voluntarily. Financial gain is a prominent incentive; the expatriates make more money than if working domestically, thus improving standards of living for their nuclear and extended families. Some employees choose to work overseas for career advancement or enriched experiences. Tangible and internal psychological rewards may provide justification for enduring current difficulties and create a buffer against environmental stressors. Moreover, some group characteristics are conducive for their adjustment to the work environment. The expatriates may not be the average employee in their respective industries and organizations. The overseas projects are viewed as highly important by the employers, with large amounts of investment as well as the country's global reputation at stake. The expatriates are typically subjected to rigorous screening during recruitment. They are likely evaluated not only for occupational or technical skills but also psychological stability and cultural and language adaptability. The employers make their best effort to select candidates who are most likely to succeed in overseas assignments. The multiple stressors and protecting factors influencing Chinese expatriates' mental health make empirical investigations on this issue more useful and significant.

This research examines the group characteristics and mental health status among a large convenience sample of Chinese expatriates. The group characteristics include gender makeup, age distributions, marital status, family structure, education, and management position. These demographic and occupational features should help us understand the personal and occupational challenges the expatriates face and the resources at their disposal for coping with the challenges. We also examine the expatriates' mental health status and its relation to their demographic and occupational characteristics. Study 1 takes a broad measure of the expatriates' current psychological distress and its relations to gender, management position and education. Study 2 investigates self-perceptions of specific symptoms of anxiety, depression, and lack of self-affirmation over the last 6 months while the expatriates are in different contexts, that is, when they are on duty, vacationing in China, or not yet deployed. By examining the current distress level and specific symptoms over a longer period of time, we aim to develop a more comprehensive understanding of the mental health of this unique group under various occupational conditions.

Data were collected from multiple samples at two large state-owned corporations working in Africa and Central Asia. The expatriates in all the samples engaged in field operations, working outdoors at the fossil-fuel exploration and extraction sites or construction areas. This type of work differs from working in factories or office buildings. All the expatriates in the samples lived in closed campuses near their worksite together with Chinese coworkers. In other words, they were relatively separated from the local communities.

STUDY 1: CHINESE EXPATRIATES' GROUP CHARACTERISTICS AND PSYCHOLOGICAL DISTRESS

This study examines the demographic and occupational characteristics and psychological distress of Chinese expatriates from various locations and analyzes the relationship between them. Based on previous U.S. research and the unique challenges confronting Chinese expatriates, we expected the expatriates to report more distress on average while working overseas compared with the norms of the general Chinese adult population. Moreover, expatriates at various worksites are faced with different working conditions and management styles and surrounded by different natural and social-cultural environments, which influence their psychological functioning. We expected to find different levels of distress among the various worksites. Meanwhile, one's adaptation to a situation is influenced by one's social and occupational roles. Men and women, manager and nonmanager, as well as workers with different education levels face different responsibilities and expectations from the families, society, and themselves. These factors may influence their perception of and response to the situation. We expected that the expatriates' psychological functioning would be influenced by gender, education and management positions.

Participants and Procedure

Seven samples of Chinese expatriates working in different sites in Africa and Central Asia were included in this study. The samples included a total number of 1,506 expatriates. The sample size from the seven sites ranged from 42 to 471. Six of the samples came from the energy sector, one from the construction industry. Chinese mental health professionals collected the data during on-site mental health workshops in Africa and Central Asia. Almost all the Chinese expatriate employees at each worksite participated in the workshops and completed the assessment materials. They filled out the questionnaires at the beginning of the workshops. They were invited (but not required) to provide their names and contact information for the purpose of facilitating follow-up services by counselors. They were assured that their responses in the surveys would remain strictly confidential.

Assessment Instruments

Participants completed the following questionnaires.

PERSONAL INFORMATION QUESTIONNAIRE

This questionnaire asks participants to indicate their gender, age, marital status, whether they have children, highest level of education, number of years working abroad, management position, as well as their names and contact information.

SYMPTOM CHECKLIST-90, CHINESE VERSION

In the original Symptom Checklist-90 (SCL-90; Derogatis, 1983), respondents rate 90 symptoms they have experienced over the last week on a 5-point scale from 1 (*none*) to 5 (*extremely serious*). The instrument yields three global indices. The Global Severity Index (GSI) is the mean score on the 90 items. In the Chinese literature, this index is often substituted with the sum of scores on the 90 items. The Positive Symptom Total (PST) is the number of items scored above one. The Positive Symptom Distress Index (PSDI) is the average score of the items scored above one. According to the author of the original scale, the symptoms fall into 10 categories, i.e., somatization, obsessive-compulsive, interpersonal sensitivity, depression, anxiety, etc. (Derogatis, 1983). The means of the scores of items in each category constitute subscale scores.

Since its translation and publication (Wang, 1984), the SCL-90 Chinese version has been used extensively in China as a measure of mental health of different community populations, including middle school and college students, teachers, doctors, nurses, workers, military personnel, ethnic minority children, and adults (see Tong, 2010 for a review). These studies generally show that the scale has good internal consistency and test–retest reliability (Chen & Li, 2003), consistent with research elsewhere (Derogatis, 2000). However, the instrument's factor structure is unclear. Chinese samples have failed to replicate the nine- or 10-factor structure proposed by the instrument's author (Feng & Zhang, 2001; Tong, 2010). This problem makes it difficult to interpret the subscale scores. Some studies have found one large factor accounting for most of the total variability, suggesting a single dimension representing global distress (Feng & Zhang, 2001). Derogatis (1983) has also suggested that the GSI is the best indicator of mental health problems. In this study, we decided to use the global indices as measures of general distress.

Despite its limitations, SCL-90, Chinese is a good choice as a comparison measure because it has been widely used in China. A national norm for the scale was published in 1986, based on 1,338 men and women from 13 provinces on mainland China (Jin, Wu, & Zhang, 1986). Subsequent Chinese studies have routinely compared their samples against this norm. In an updated national norm based on a sample of 1,890 community adults from 21 provinces (Tong, 2010), the GSI and most subscale scores were close to the 1986 norm. We compared the expatriates' global indices against the published Chinese national norms where the data are available, though our main focus is on the relationship between the expatriates' psychological distress and demographic and occupational characteristics.

Results

DEMOGRAPHIC AND OCCUPATIONAL CHARACTERISTICS

These data came from the Personal Information Questionnaire.

Gender imbalance. A total of 1,505 respondents indicated their gender in the questionnaire. Among them 92.43% were men and 7.57% were women. The men had longer tenures on overseas assignments, with a mean of 4.50 years and standard deviation of 3.23 years, ranging from less than one up to 18 years, whereas the women on average had worked overseas for 3.0 years, with a standard deviation of 2.50 years, ranging from less than one up to 12 years.

Different age distributions between men and women. Participants' ages were coded into four intervals, that is, 20 to 29, 30 to 39, 40 to 49, and 50 and above. Among the men, the two largest age groups were those between 30 and 39 and those between 40 and 49 years, jointly accounting for approximately 80% of the men in the samples (Table 1). Approximately 80% of the men were in their first marriages and more than 77% had children (Table 2). The majority of the men were at the prime of their lives; this cohort

TABLE 1 Age Distribution of Male and Female Expatriates, Studies 1 and 2

	Study 1		Study 2	
	Men ($n = 1391$)	Women ($n = 114$)	Men ($n = 4227$)	Women ($n = 144$)
20–29	15.7%	49.2%	20.98%	25.69%
30–39	38.6%	14.9%	39.58%	30.56%
40–49	39.8%	28.9%	25.81%	24.31%
50 +	3.6%	2.6%	3.52%	4.86%
No response	2.3%	4.4%	10.10%	14.58%

TABLE 2 Marriage and Children, Studies 1 and 2

	Study 1		Study 2	
	Men ($n = 1391$)	Women ($n = 114$)	Men ($n = 4227$)	Women ($n = 144$)
In first marriage	78.00%	43.86%	78.64%	63.89%
Never married	11.72%	30.70%	17.06%	29.17%
Other[a]	2.08%	2.63%	2.86%	6.94%
No response	8.20%	22.81%	1.44%	0%
With children	75.56%	37.72%	60.75%	52.78%
No children	21.78%	59.65%	22.64%	27.08%
No response	2.66%	2.63%	16.61%	20.14%

[a]This category includes those who are divorced, remarried, widowed, etc.

is likely to be the backbones of the work force in their companies. Meanwhile, they are going through a period in their lives characterized with multiple responsibilities to their spouses, children, and aging parents. On the other hand, the number of women peaked in the age groups between 20 and 29 (accounting for nearly 50% of all female respondents). The second largest age group for women was between 40 and 49 (accounting for approximately 29% of all female respondents). The percentage of women between 30 and 39 was smaller than that of men. This is the age interval when most Chinese women are raising young children. A smaller percentage (approximately 52%) of the women were married compared to their male colleagues. These results are consistent with the traditional gender roles in China; men spend their most vigorous years working outside home, even in foreign countries far away from family if necessary. On the other hand, women are less likely to work far away from family once they marry and have children (especially young children). Only a small fraction of the men and women were age 50 or older.

Level of education and management positions. The men and women had higher levels of education compared with the general Chinese population. More specifically, 72.67% of the men and 90% of the women had completed junior college or above. For management positions, 40.35% of men and 24.04% of women identified themselves as managers. The fact that the women had higher education but lower positions in the organizational hierarchy suggests the women faced more formidable career challenges than the men.

Psychological distress and demographic/occupational characteristics. We compared the global indices of the men and women against the Chinese national norms where published data were available. We also examined the influences of management position, education, age, and length of overseas assignment on psychological distress. Other demographic characteristics such as whether they are married or have children are not included in the analyses, because these variables are closely related to age; the youngest groups are most likely to be unmarried and childless.

Gender effects. Overall, the women had significantly higher Global Symptom Index (GSI), $t(1464) = 2.95$, $p < 0.01$, Positive Symptom Totals (PST), $t(1464) = 2.56$, $p = 0.01$, and Positive Symptom Distress Index (PSDI), $t(1422) = 2.14$, $p < 0.05$ than the men. This result is unsurprising considering the women's minority status and the challenges they faced in career development.

Comparisons with national norms and between sites. The national norms of 1988 and 2010 found no gender difference on the global indices. The means of our male and female expatriate samples across different worksites on the GSI and PST were higher than the unisex national norms (Table 3), which did not report PSDI.

We examined the differences among the seven worksites on GSI, PST, and PSDI. The results reported below are based on data from the men. Including the women in the analyses did not change the results significantly. Because of the small number of women, it would be inappropriate to compare them across different worksites separately. One-way analysis of variance (ANOVA) indicate significant differences among the seven worksites on the GSI, $F(6, 1309) = 7.70$, $p < 0.001$. Four sites showed lower mean scores, whereas three sites showed higher mean scores than the 1988 and 2006 national norms. The seven sites also showed significant differences on the PST, $F(6, 1349) = 8.20$, $p < 0.001$. All seven sites reported more symptoms than the 1986 national norm. Meanwhile, the differences among the sites were large. There was also significant differences on PSDI, $F(6, 1309) = 2.64$, $p = 0.01$ among the sites.

Influence of management position. The expatriates who self-identified as managers reported higher levels of distress as measured in the GSI than those self-identified as nonmanagers, $t(1451) = 3.12$, $p < 0.01$. The managers

TABLE 3 Symptom Checklist-90 Global Indices of Male and Female Expatriates in Comparison to Published National Norms, Study 1

		GSI		PST		PSDI	
	N	*M*	*SD*	*M*	*SD*	*M*	*SD*
1986 national norm	1338	129.96	38.76	24.92	18.41	—	—
2006 national norm	1890	130.02	33.63	—	—	—	—
Expatriate female	109	143.24	43.99	37.20	23.35	2.34	0.40
Expatriate male	1357	131.62	39.31	31.50	22.33	2.26	0.37

GSI = Global Severity Index, PST = Positive Symptom Total, PSDI = Positive Symptom Distress Index.

also had a larger number of positive symptoms, as measured in the PST, $t(1451) = 4.56$, $p < 0.01$. The managers and nonmanagers did not differ in the PSDI, $p > 0.05$. These results were based on men and women; excluding the women from the analyses did not change the results significantly.

Mental health and education. We assigned numerical values to the expatriates' levels of education and treated it as a continuous variable. We used the values of 1, 2, 3, and 4 to represent the four levels of education, that is., high school or below, two-year college, four-year college, and graduate school. We calculated the correlation between level of education and GSI, PSI, and PSID. Education had a significant positive correlation with GSI, $r = 0.88$ and PSI, $r = 0.10$, $ps < 0.01$. The expatriates with higher levels of education had more severe symptoms overall and reported larger numbers of positive symptoms. The correlation between education and PSDI was not significant, $r = 0.02$, $p > 0.05$, a result likely due to the restricted range of PSDI; the respondents' positive symptoms were all relatively mild. The above results were based on both men and women; excluding the women from the analyses did not change the results significantly.

Age effect. Because men and women had different patterns of age distribution and the samples of women were extremely small, we excluded women when examining the age effect on mental health. We do not have enough women in the samples to compare them across different age groups. One-way ANOVA indicates that men in the four age groups did not differ on any of the global measures of distress, $ps > 0.05$.

Length of overseas assignment. The correlation between length of overseas assignment and mental health status among the men and women were not significant, $ps > 0.05$. Excluding women from the analyses did not change the results significantly.

STUDY 2: SYMPTOMS IN CONTEXT: ON DUTY, VACATIONING, AND PREDEPLOYMENT EXPATRIATES

Study 1 examined the expatriates' current distress while stationed overseas and its relations to demographic and occupational characteristics. Expatriates' assignments last for certain periods of time, ranging from months to years. They go through different phases in adjusting to their overseas environment (Black & Mendenhall, 1991; Black, Mendenhall, & Oddou, 1991). Point-in-time measures such as those taken in Study 1 may not capture the variations over the course of their overseas assignments. The transition from the home-country environment to active deployment overseas is likely to pose considerable psychological challenge. On the other hand, vacations at home provide the opportunity for rest, reunification with family, and returning to a familiar environment. In Study 2 we take a more dynamic approach to understanding the expatriates' psychological adjustment by comparing their functioning in different contexts, that is, after accepting assignments but before deployment (predeployment), while working over-seas (on duty) and vacationing in home country (vacationing). If the difficult-ies associated with overseas assignments are responsible for the expatriates' negative responses, then those currently on duty should show exacerbated symptoms relative to their vacationing and predeployment colleagues. The vacationing and predeployment expatriates make appropriate control groups for those on duty because all three groups have been subjected to the same screening and accepted the same assignments. Moreover, Study 2 examines the expatriates' self-perception of specific symptoms of depression, anxiety, and lack of self-affirmation over a longer period of time, that is, the last 6 months. These measures provide more fine-grained understanding of the expatriates' symptom profiles. As in Study 1, we examine the influence of gender, management position, and education on mental health.

Participants and Procedure

Participants were 4,436 employees working for one of the Chinese state-owned companies in Study 1 with assignments in various sites in Africa and Central Asia. The on duty expatriates completed the surveys in the same way as in Study 1. Vacationing and predeployment expatriates completed the surveys during mental health trainings at a facility in China. The worksites of the participants were not consistently recorded as in Study 1.

Assessment Instruments

PERSONAL INFORMATION QUESTIONNAIRE

This instrument was the same as in Study 1.

GENERAL-HEALTH QUESTIONNAIRE, CHINESE

We used an instrument developed by Li and Kam (2002) based on a Chinese translation of the 30-item General Health Questionnaire (GHQ; Chan & Chan, 1983), which in turn originated from Goldberg's 60-item GHQ (Vieweg & Hedlund, 1983). Li and Kam (2002) eliminated 10 items from the 30-item GHQ that were ambiguous in Chinese due to linguistic and cultural differ-ences, leaving 20 items with positive and negative valences that fall into three broad categories, that is, anxiety (six items), depression (five items), and a group they labeled "self-affirmation" (nine items). We moved one item from their self-affirmation scale to depression scale because it has a clear reference to depression ("feeling unhappy or depressed"), thus yielding six items for depression and eight items for self-affirmation. The anxiety and depression scales consist of items commonly linked to those negative emotions. The self-affirmation scale consists of items related with self-esteem and positive affect. They conducted two factor analyses studies with a total of 1,142 college students confirming the factor structure. A subsequent factor analyses study confirmed the factor structure of this instrument (Li & Wei, 2007). Meanwhile, the GHQ family of instruments has received wide support as reliable and valid measures of mental health. We believe these items serve as valid measures of anxiety, depression and self-affirmation.

For each item, participants indicated whether they had had the experience within the last 6 months by checking "yes" or "no," which were then assigned the numerical values of one or zero. We computed the subscale scores for anxiety, depression, and self-affirmation. Higher anxiety and depression scores mean more symptoms (i.e., worse adjustment), whereas higher self-affirmation scores indicate more positive affect and higher self esteem (i.e., better adjustment).

Results

DEMOGRAPHIC AND OCCUPATIONAL CHARACTERISTICS

Gender imbalance. Women were even more under-represented in this sample than in Study 1. A total of 4,371 respondents indicated their gender in the questionnaires. Among them 96.7% were men and only 3.3% were women. Among the employees who had worked overseas (i.e., the on duty and vacationing expatriates) and reported their length of overseas assignment, the men ($n = 3,289$) had longer overseas tenures than their female colleagues. On average the men had worked for 4.83 years on overseas assignments, with a standard deviation of 3.03 years, ranging from less than one year up to 22 years. The women ($n = 55$) on average had worked overseas for 3.94 years, with a standard deviation of 3.20 years, ranging from less than one year up to 13 years.

Age distributions. As in Study 1, only a small fraction of men and women were age 50 years or older (Table 1). Among the men, the largest age group consisted of those between 30 and 39 years, followed by those between 20 and 29 and between 40 and 49 (Table 1). As in Study 1, most of the men were in their first marriages and had children (Table 2). Women's age distribution was more comparable to the men's than in Study 1 (Table 2). Consistent with Study 1, smaller percentages of women were married and with children than men, but these gender differences were smaller than in Study 1.

Education and management positions. As in Study 1, men and women had more education than the general population, with 71.61% of the men and

90.28% of the women having completed at least junior college. Moreover, 33.10% of the men and 30.56% of the women identified themselves as managers. The proportions of men and women in management positions were more equitable than in Study 1.

EXPATRIATE CHARACTERISTICS AND SYMPTOMS

Gender differences. None of the differences between men and women on the GHQ-20 scores reached statistical significance. The means of the women on all the GHQ-20 scores were higher than that of the men, a pattern different from Study 1.

Context, management position, and symptoms. We examined how managers and nonmanagers fared on the GHQ-20 anxiety, depression, and self-affirmation scores across different contexts, i.e., on duty, vacationing and predeployment.

Anxiety. A two by three ANOVA with the expatriates' position (managers vs. nonmanagers) and context (on duty, vacationing, and predeployment) as between group factors and anxiety score as the dependent variable revealed a significant main effect of context, $F(2, 4290) = 47.15$, $p < 0.001$; on duty, vacationing, and predeployment expatriates reported different levels of anxiety. Planned contrasts revealed that on duty expatriates were more anxious than their vacationing and predeployment colleagues combined, $t(4293) = -8.93$, $p < 0.001$, whereas the later two groups did not differ from each other, $t(4293) = -1.32$, $p > 0.05$. There was no main effect for position, $F(1, 4290) = 1,87$, $p > 0.05$. Overall, managers did not differ significantly from nonmanagers in anxiety. However, there was a significant interaction between context and position, $F(2, 4290) = 3.05$, $p < 0.05$, indicating that the pattern of differences among on duty, vacationing, and predeployment expatriates differed between managers and nonmanagers. We compared the managers' and nonmanagers' anxiety scores across the different contexts (Table 4). Among the predeployment expatriates, the difference

TABLE 4 General Health Questionnaire-20 Scores of Nonmanagers and Managers in Different Contexts, Study 2

	Nonmanagers						Managers					
	On Duty			Vacationing			Predeparture			On Duty			Vacationing			Predeparture		
	N	M	SD	N	M	SD	N	M	SD	N	M	SD	N	M	SD	N	M	SD
Anxiety	2129	2.07	2.00	474	1.56	1.77	242	1.48	1.77	1015	2.48	2.07	367	1.71	1.88	69	1.35	1.56
Depression	2129	1.14	1.50	474	0.56	1.08	242	0.67	1.20	1015	1.22	1.54	367	0.60	1.10	69	0.43	0.87
Self-affirmation	2126	5.47	2.15	474	5.91	1.84	242	5.83	1.81	1014	5.24	2.20	367	5.89	1.89	69	6.32	1.80

between managers and nonmanagers was not significant, $t(309) = 0.58$, $p > 0.05$. However, the on duty managers were significantly more anxious than the nonmanagers, $t(3142) = 5.37$, $p < 0.01$. The managers and nonmanagers did not differ from each other on any of the GHQ-20 scores while on vacation, $p > 0.05$. This pattern of results indicate that though managers and nonmanagers became more anxious while working overseas relative to when they were vacationing or prior to their deployment, the managers suffered greater increases in anxiety while onsite.

Depression. A two by three ANOVA with the expatriates' position (managers vs. nonmanagers) and context (on duty, vacationing, and predeployment) as between group factors and depression score as the dependent variable revealed a significant main effect of context, $F(2, 4290) = 70.11$, $p < 0.001$; on duty, vacationing, and predeployment expatriates reported different levels of depression. Planned contrasts revealed that on duty expatriates fared worse than their vacationing and predeployment colleagues combined, $t(4293) = -10.68$, $p < 0.01$, whereas the later two groups did not differ from each other $t(4293) = 0.48$, $p > 0.05$. There was no main effect for position, $F(1, 4290) = 0.28$, $p > 0.05$, or interaction between position and context, $F(1, 4290) = 1.31$, $p > .05$, indicating that the pattern of changes across the contexts we examined (predeployment, vacationing and on duty) did not differ between the managers and nonmanagers (Table 4).

Self-affirmation. A two by three ANOVA with the expatriates' position (managers vs. nonmanagers) and context (on duty, vacationing, and predeployment) as between group factors and self-affirmation score as the dependent variable revealed a significant main effect of context, $F(2, 4290) = 30.22$, $p < 0.001$; on duty, vacationing, and predeployment expatriates reported different levels of self-affirmation. Planned contrasts revealed that on duty expatriates fared worse than their vacationing and predeployment colleagues combined, $t(4293) = -6.72$, $p < 0.01$, whereas the later two groups did not differ from each other $t(4293) = -0.28$, $p > 0.05$. There was no main effect for position, $F(1, 4290) = 0.59$, $p > 0.05$. However, there was a significant interaction between position and context, $F(1, 4290) = 3.39$, $p < 0.05$, indicating that managers differed from nonmanagers across the contexts we examined (predeployment, vacationing, and on duty; Table 4). Planned contrast revealed that predeployment managers reported more positive self-affirmation than predeployment nonmanagers, $t(309) = -1.99$, $p < 0.05$, but on duty managers reported lower levels of self-affirmation than on duty nonmanagers, $t(3142) = 2.71$, $p < 0.01$.

Influence of education. The expatriates' level of education had a strong and significant negative correlation with self-affirmation, $r = -0.75$, $p < 0.01$, indicating that the higher the expatriates' level of education, the less happy they were. Education had no significant correlation with anxiety or depression.

GENERAL DISCUSSIONS

The two studies reported in this article have examined the mental health of Chinese expatriates in the energy and construction sectors in Africa and Central Asia and its relations to some group characteristics. For mental health, we have examined distress while the expatriates were on duty (Study 1) as well as specific symptoms of anxiety, depression, and lack of self-affirmation across different contexts, that is, when they were on duty, vacationing and prior to being deployed (Study 2).

Several demographic and occupational characteristics make this group unique among the Chinese working population. The expatriates were overwhelmingly male, at their prime ages and better educated than the general population, giving the impression that their jobs are demanding and stereotypically suited for energetic, competent, and hardy men. Most of the men and more than one half of the women were married with children. This is a group that faces multiple and sometimes conflicting expectations and responsibilities from their social and occupational roles.

In Study 1, the expatriates on average reported more distress symptoms while working overseas than the general Chinese population. In Study 2, the expatriates' anxiety, depression, and lack of self-affirmation worsened when working overseas compared with when they were not yet deployed or taking vacations. These results are consistent with the challenges they face while stationed overseas. On the other hand, Study 1 also shows that the expatriates' average distress symptoms were mild, that is, between 2 (*light*) and 3 (*medium*; Table 3) on a 1 to 5 scale. The expatriates' average levels of anxiety, depression and self-affirmation in Study 2 confirmed this result. Moreover, Study 2 shows that when the expatriates were taking vacations, their anxiety, depression, and self-affirmation returned to predeployment baseline levels, suggesting that the distress they experienced at the worksites were temporary and reversible. We believe this pattern reflects the expatriates' resilience; they were able to cope with the stress on the worksite, keep negative responses to a low level and recover quickly once the stressors were removed.

Study 1 shows that expatriates working in different sites varied in distress level, presumably as a result of different management style, social, and natural conditions. Despite the regional diversity, consistent patterns have emerged in the expatriates' mental health in relation to their demographic and occupational characteristics. These include the influences of management positions, education and context (whether they are on duty, vacationing, or predeployment) on mental health.

Management Position

In Study 1, managers reported more distress than nonmanagers while working overseas. Study 2 provides a glimpse into the time-course of the managers' and nonmanagers' adjustment from predeployment to during-deployment and while on vacation. Managers and nonmanagers were more anxious and depressed with lower self-affirmation while working overseas compared with when vacationing or before deployment. However, the managers suffered a larger increase in anxiety and decrease in self-affirmation from pre- to postdeployment than nonmanagers. When they accepted the assignment but before taking positions overseas, the managers had started with higher self-affirmation and less anxiety. This reaction suggests that managers had higher expectations for their overseas experiences and were more excited about the opportunities. However, they became more anxious and self-doubting than their subordinates while working overseas. This is probably due to their multiple responsibilities and heavier work overload. Managers work harder and have more issues to worry about and resolve than their subordinates. The harsh realities on the ground may lead to a stronger sense of disappointment among the managers.

Education

More educated expatriates reported more distress (Study 1) and lower self-affirmation (Study 2). This might be due to two reasons. First, education is associated with management positions. The managers, who have higher responsibility, workload, and stress are more likely to have higher education. Second, more educated people have higher expectation for their lives. They are more likely to be disappointed while working overseas.

Gender

Women's minority position in the overseas worksites makes their psychological adjustment an important issue of concern. However, the data on expatriate women's mental health from Studies 1 and 2 are somewhat inconsistent. In Study 1, women reported greater current distress. However, in Study 2, women fared at least as well as the men on self-perceptions of anxiety, depression, and self-affirmation. This inconsistency reflects the multiple factors influencing women's adjustment on overseas assignments. On the one hand, some societal factors make it more challenging for women to successfully adjust to their overseas assignments than men. Taking overseas assignments is incompatible with the traditional role of women, resulting in conflict between their occupational responsibilities and obligations to families. Working in harsh environments in Africa and Central Asia in the energy and construction industries exacerbates this role conflict.

Moreover, women may face considerable barriers in their career develop-ment overseas, as suggested by their higher levels of education but lower proportion of managers as a group in Study 1. These factors may have led women to complain more strongly in Study 1. On the other hand, difficulties for women to work overseas may have led employers to deploy women only after thorough evaluations. Meanwhile, presumably female employees would be particularly cautious in taking overseas assignments. This selection and self-selection process may have contributed to women's minority status. The women who have received and accepted overseas assignments may be considered as an elite group; presumably the women and their employers/ supervisors believe they are psychologically prepared for their tasks. This rationale is plausible given the fact that in Study 2 women were smaller in proportion than in Study 1 but adjusted as well as their male colleagues. However, the small number of women in the samples limit our ability to draw firm conclusions.

CONCLUSIONS AND SUGGESTIONS

With the rapid increase in China's overseas investment and economic activi-ties (e.g., French, 2014), mental health needs in the expatriate Chinese com-munity have become significant and real. These needs are more pronounced than among the general population and call for systematic workplace behavioral health interventions such as Employee Assistance Programs. The results of this study suggest the following directions for employers, man-agers, and clinicians to help expatriates adapt to their overseas assignments.

Family Support

Most expatriates (especially the men) are in their first marriages and with children. Family is important part of their core value systems. Quantitative data collected by clinicians indicate that the top-listed worries and concerns for the expatriates were related with spouse relations, parental care and child-rearing. It is important to support expatriates' relations and communi-cations with families at all stages of their assignments, that is, before deployment, while on duty, visiting home, and after repatriation. Support for the expatriates' spouses, children, and parents would also be useful for maintaining the integrity of their family system and success on their overseas assignments (Black & Stevens, 1989).

Onsite Support and Vacations

Providing regular and accessible mental health care at or close to the worksites would help expatriates manage stress, relieve negative emotions, and increase resilience. Ensuring that expatriates have adequate vacation time will also be essential for the expatriates to maintain family connections, recuperate, and maintain long-term mental health.

Managers' Health

Managers face greater stress because of higher responsibilities and expectations from outside and inside, hence bigger challenges in adjustment and adaptation. Study 2 indicates that managers suffer greater deterioration in mental health while working overseas from the predeployment stage. Employers and mental health professionals may help reduce this deterioration with more thorough training and education before deployment overseas to help managers develop objective understanding of the situation on the ground, better prepare for the challenges, and avoid a sense of disappointment and helplessness.

Limitations of the Study and Future Research Directions

Because the data came from convenience samples, we cannot be certain that they are representative of the Chinese expatriates in the energy and construction sectors in Africa and Central Asia. More systematic research is needed to obtain an objective understanding of the group characteristics and mental health status of this population. Moreover, the measures of mental health were not truly diagnostic but consist of symptom counts. More systematic approaches will be needed for firm and clear assessments of the expatriates' mental health status. Finally, as in most research conducted in applied settings, we cannot isolate the causes of the differences in mental health observed in the expatriate samples with certainty given our methodology. Despite of these limitations, this is the first empirical study with a large sample size on the emerging issues of Chinese expatriates' mental health, thus making it noteworthy.

REFERENCES

Black, J. S., & Gregersen, H. B. (1999). The right way to manage expats. *Harvard Business Review, 77,* 52–62.

Black, J. S., & Mendenhall, M. (1991). The u-curve adjustment hypothesis revisited: A review and theoretical framework. *Journal of International Business Studies, 22,* 225–247.

Black, J. S., Mendenhall, M., & Oddou, G. (1991). Toward a comprehensive model of international adjustment: An integration of multiple theoretical perspectives. *Academy of Management Review, 16,* 292–317.

Black, J. S., & Stevens, G. K. (1989). The influence of the spouse on American expatriate adjustment and intent to stay in Pacific Rim overseas assignments. *Journal of Management, 15,* 529–544.

Brautigam, D. (2011). Chinese development assistance to Africa. *East Asia Forum*. Retrieved from http://www.eastasiaforum.org/2011/12/25/chinese-development-aid-in-africa/

Chan, D., & Chan, T. (1983). Reliability, validity and the structure of the General Health Questionnaire in a Chinese context. *Psychological Medicine, 13*, 363–371.

Chen, S., & Li, L. (2003). SCL-90 Xin Du Xiao Du Jian Yan He Chang Mo De Zai Bi Jiao [Evaluation of the reliability and validity of SCL-90 and re-comparison of its norms]. *Zhong Guo Jing Shen Shen Jing Ji Bing Zha Zhi [Chinese Journal of Psychiatric and Neurological Disorders], 29*, 323–327.

Derogatis, L. R. (1983). *SCL-90-R administration, scoring & procedures manual-II*. Towson, MD: Clinical Psychometric Research.

Derogatis, L. R. (2000) Symptom Checklist-90-Revised. In A. J. Rush, M. M. First, & D. Blacker (Eds.), *Handbook of psychiatric measures* (pp. 81–84). Washington, DC: American Psychiatric Association.

Feng, Z., & Zhang, D. (2001). Zhong Guo Ban SCL-90 Xiao Du Yan Jiu [Study on the validity of the Symptom Check-List-90, Chinese version]. *Di San Jun Yi Da Xue Xue Bao [Acta Academiae Medicine Militaris Tertiae], 23*, 481–483.

French, H. (2014). *China's second continent: How a million migrants are building a new empire in Africa*. New York, NY: Knopf.

Jin, H., Wu, W., & Zhang, M. (1986). Zhong Guo Zheng Chang Ren SCL-90 Ping Ding Jie Guo De Chu Bu Fen Xi [Preliminary analyses of the results of assessment with SCL-90 in Chinese normal population]. *Zhong Gou Shen Jing Ji Bing Za Zhi [Chinese Journal of Neurological Disorders], 12*, 260–263.

Li, H., & Kam, W. B. (2002). Ce Liang Da Xue Sheng De Xin Li Wenti: GHQ-20 De Jie Gou Ji Qi Xin Du He Xiao Du [Assessing psychological well-being of college student: psychometric properties of GHQ-20]. *Xin Li Fa Zhan Yu Jiao Yu [Psychological Development and Education], 18*, 75–79.

Li, Y., & Wei, Y. (2007). Yi Ban Jian Kang Wen Juan (GHQ-20) Zai Da Xue Sheng Zhong De Xin Xiao Du Jian Yan [The psychometric properties of GHQ-20 in university students]. *Zhong Guo Jian Kang Xin Li Xue Za Zhi [China Journal of Health Psychology], 15*, 11–13

Piao, Y. (2006). Zhong Guo Dui Fei Zhou Zhi Jie Tou Zi De Fa Zhan Li Cheng Yu Wei Lai Qu Shi [The evolution and future trend of China's direct investment in Africa]. *Hai Wai Tou Zi Yu Chu Kou Xin Dai [Overseas investment and export credit]*. Retrieved from http://www.eximbank.gov.cn/topic/hwtz/2006/1_19.doc

Sun, Y. (2014). Africa in China's foreign policy. *The Brookings Institute*. Retrieved from http://www.brookings.edu/~/media/research/files/papers/2014/04/africa-china-policy-sun/africa-in-china-web_cmg7.pdf

Tong, H. (2010). SCL-90 Liang Biao Ji Qi Chang Mo 20 Nian Bian Qian Zhi Yan Jiu [Research on the SCL-90 and changes to its norms over the last 20 years]. *Xin Li Ke Xue [Psychological Science], 33*, 928–930.

Truman, S. D., Sharar, D. A., & Pompe, J. C. (2011). The mental health status of expatriate versus U.S. domestic workers: A comparative study. *International Journal of Mental Health, 40*, 3–18.

Vieweg, B. W., & Hedlund, J. L. (1983). The General Health Questionnaire (GHQ): A comprehensive review. *Journal of Operational Psychiatry, 14,* 74–81.

Wang, Z. (1984). Zheng Zhuang Zi Ping Liang Biao SCL-90 [Symptom Checklist SCL-90]. *Shang Hai Jing Shen Yi Xue [Shanghai Psychiatry], 2,* 68–70.

Yi, Y. (2011). China probes its Africa model. *China Dialogue.* Retrieved from http://www.chinadialogue.net/article/show/single/en/4470-Chinaprobes-its-Africa-model-1

Index

Printed and bound by CPI Group (UK) Ltd, Croydon, CR0 4YY

21/10/2024

01777095-0009